JESSICA DUEMIG

WARRIOR

CHALLENGE ACCEPTED

WARRIOR

FOR MY #MySaintlyParents

I love you and I could not have done it without you.

But seriously, thank God I had a two-bedroom condo.

A Letter to the Reader

Dear reader, you wonderful, strong human:

I never considered myself to be overtly feminine. I grew up playing soccer, and I was good. I had a solid build, killer quads and the obligatory ponytail. I was strong. I was invincible and I was all-sports, all the time. I believed in function over form; and I didn't have time for fashion. If there were ever two things I hung my tiara on, they were my eyelashes and my boobs. I always had super long lashes – enviable if I do say so myself…And man, I had good boobs. They were round and perky – they protruded, rather than scooping if you know what I mean, and with the right bra, oh the cleavage. They fit my body, were fairly symmetrical and completely natural with just the right amount of salon-induced tan. This introduction may sound conceited. I call it nostalgic. In November of 2016, I found a lump in my left breast that would ultimately change my life.

As I wrote this book, I found myself stopping every few pages, contemplating why I was doing so… I'm not special. I don't know why what I think and experienced seems worth putting out there; but then I realized that I essentially wrote the guidebook that I wish I had when I was first diagnosed. You'll come to read about all the questions from the doctors and social workers regarding whether or not I wanted a support group or to talk to someone in my *same exact shoes*. And I didn't. Not in the traditional sense, but more specifically because I didn't consider any of the 'supporters' that the hospital referred me to as being in my *same exact shoes*.

Sure, they had cancer; breast cancer. But they didn't have triple negative, metaplastic breast cancer. They were in their 30s, but not 32. Not single and unattached. Not without child(ren). Not with 60-hour-a-week corporate jobs where they were the only woman in management. Not living alone in Miami. Again, I'm not special, I'm just underrepresented. In the same way I don't pretend to understand how on earth I would have explained my situation to my child, I don't know how speaking with any of these women would have helped me. Maybe that's unfair. Maybe I don't care. Hey look! I'm a poet and I didn't even know it! Take the laughs where you can get them, folks!

This book will take you through the nine most challenging months of my (now) 35 years on this earth. This isn't a bitching session about a terrible predicament. It's not an epic tale of finding love in the middle of a category five shitstorm. It's a raw, real, uncensored, (hopefully) uplifting journey that you'll take with me through the hard times, the weird stuff, real life, the triumph and the *what the fuck do I do now*.

As you read, please don't feel bad about laughing at or with me. After all, if we can't laugh about it, we'll cry, *amiright*? Be warned: You'll probably come to learn way TMI about Jessie Poo, and you may at times think I'm full of shit. (You could be right (#SelfAware); but not about this.) Unlike a lot of the commercials you see on TV, breast cancer is not always a pink-shirted, middle-aged woman with a husband and a dog, who reads the morning paper and goes for long hikes. It's also not a my-life-is-over-let-me-just-park-it-by-the-toilet-and-puke-my-day-away death sentence.

My story is one of a single, career-driven, pre-kid, badass woman living alone in one of the most superficial cities in the world, who takes no shit from anyone. This is my journey; one I went into relatively blind. I hadn't seen family members deal with this. I didn't have friends who lived to tell the tale. I don't pretend to know how someone in a different life situation would have handled some of the things I went through, but you're going to read about how *I* dealt with it. How *I* got through it. How *I* survived it. I hope you'll find my story to be an entertaining one; but also, a real one that you'll relate to on one level or another and possibly even share with someone who can benefit from the overall message.

Best of luck in the battle of and for your life! Give it hell.

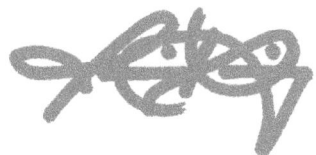

PART I

PHYSICAL

CHAPTER
ONE

PART I: BEFORE YOU CONTINUE

Please remember as you read through these anecdotes, that **I am not a doctor**. I completed exactly one science course in college and went to Business School...not Medical School. I am providing information as *I* understood it, based on *my* specific case, and *my* comfort level with *my* doctors. If you take anything from this book, let it be this: **YOU KNOW YOUR BODY BETTER THAN ANYONE ELSE.** And it is, indeed, **YOUR** body. As I write about all the decisions 'we' made, I say it in solidarity with my own sanity and in concert with my doctors.

I decided to have a bi-lateral (double) mastectomy as opposed to a lumpectomy or a unilateral (single) mastectomy. *I decided* to use silicone versus saline implants, and to use the textured, round, gummy bear variety instead of a smooth, teardrop. *I decided* to have a chemo port inserted during surgery, rather than taking the chemicals through my veins. And *I decided* to push for a shorter overall duration of chemo, rather than extending it by a couple of months to give my body more time to recover in between infusions.

Any single one of those decisions could have been altered, and maybe I would have had a similar recovery. Maybe not. Either way, I knew my body – maybe better than I had ever wanted to – and it was/is mine. And yours is yours. Take my stories and experiences – as well as my definitions and understanding of the terms – and allow the information to enhance your decision-making process. **That's it.**

CHAPTER
TWO

SPOILER ALERT: I'M FINE

It was November of 2016. The Jets were decent (5-4 to that point in the season). University of South Florida football was kicking ass with a record of 9-2 and Southern Miss was being very *Southern Miss* with a record of 5-6 despite a great season the year prior. Bowl Week[1] was just around the corner and I was re-discovering my love for soccer #HalaMadrid. I was about six months into a new job as an Account Director for a sports broadcasting network at a global advertising agency in Miami and life was good. My sister, Dianne, and I had finalized our plans for her 30th birthday trip to Scandinavia for January 2017 and The Hallmark Channel was about to

---

[1] I was contracted for the ninth year in a row to produce ESPN's Gasparilla Bowl from Tropicana Field in St. Petersburg, FL

start their Countdown to Christmas (seriously – is there anything better than that??)

My family was healthy and happy, my grandparents were in good shape, I had a solid group of friends and was debating getting a dog for, like, the 100th time. NOTE: I did not get a dog, but instead, settled for an orchid. It was dead within 2 weeks. Lucky dog.

And then I woke up. I mean, literally woke up to a dull, but concentrated pain. I'm a side sleeper – I think. I mean who knows; I sleep alone, so there was no one to confirm it. All I know is I start on one side and wake up on the other. The in-between remains a mystery. Either way, that day, I woke up on my left side. The pain wasn't intense, but it was there, poking me in the boob. After a little bit of self-examination, I diagnosed myself as being dramatic and went on with my day.

And then I woke up. About a month later, not quite Christmas, but the week before. It was Bowl Week and I was at a hotel in St. Petersburg – Florida, not Russia – and my little nodule of drama was back wreaking havoc. What I thought was a minor pimple or ingrown hair a month ago, was now more pronounced, seemingly gelatinous and about the size of a gumball. Not the giant gumballs that were totally worth a quarter on their own, but more like the ½ size ones that lost their flavor within seconds. Not good. But Aunt Flow was in town, so I chalked it up to my menstrual cycle and went about my day.

Something wasn't right though, and deep down I knew it. Walking through Downtown St. Pete, full of tacos at that moment, I called to make an appointment with my Primary Care Physician (PCP) for the week between Christmas and New Year's. Flash forward, Bowl Week completed its annual quota of EPIC, Christmas was awesome and chock full of gluttony, this Christmas's #SeasonalSelfie[2] was old-school Christmas light bulb necklaces with fancy head bands; and, just like that, I was back in the 305.

The University of Miami – formerly, the bane of my existence, growing up a Florida State Seminoles fan – was now the place that I relied on for general healthcare needs. I find that usually when I make an appointment with the doctor, my ailment mysteriously goes away the day before I'm set to see the doctor...I know I'm not alone in that, but still, every time, I feel like a moron. *I promise, it was happening just last night.* Today was not one of those days. The doctor confirmed that she felt the same lump, but she was sure *it was nothing.* She sent me for a mammogram and ultrasound anyway.

It's amazing how quickly appointments materialize when there's even the slightest fear of something really bad. Maybe it's the potential windfall of insurance funds; maybe they actually have the patient's best interest/health in

---

[2] My family started taking 'Seasonal Selfies' earlier that year at Easter time, realizing that we needed more fun, all-inclusive family photos. Each holiday, a member of the immediate family chooses a set of matching accessories that we adorn during the celebration and take a selfie. The tradition is still going strong!

mind…I choose to think it's the latter. Either way, I was into the radiology department within the first week of January for both tests.

The mammogram confirmed what seemed like two (!!) masses in my left breast; and something funky in my right (again, !!). My words, not theirs. The ultrasound took a closer, different look. You know it is not a great situation when they utilize the fancy doctor network of global on-call analysts to read the scans. My doctor was in Australia; no accent though #Bummer. He proceeded to tell me that he could confirm the 'two' masses in my left breast, and that there was indeed something going on on the right side too. He concluded that they were most likely fluid-filled cysts and nothing to worry about. He scheduled me for an aspiration of the two 'cysts' in my left breast and a biopsy of whatever was in my right breast within the week.

A quick Public Service Announcement: It is never too early to start checking yourself for Breast Cancer. Unfortunately, Breast Cancer – especially Triple Negative Breast Cancer – is becoming more and more common in younger and younger people, and when caught early, can be treated quickly without too much interference in your life. If you do the checks – there are a number of resources if you are unsure how to do it – and find anything that seems a little off, go get a mammogram, or at least to see your Primary Care Physician. I'm sure people will tell you that mammograms are really painful, but trust me when I tell you, the alternative is or can be much, much worse.

Also, while *maybe* uncomfortable, my mammogram didn't actually hurt that bad. I know everyone has a different pain tolerance, but seriously, make like a Nike commercial, and *Just Do It.*

Our Scandinavia trip was 2 weeks away, and I was laying on a surgical table, with a squishy fish in one hand and a solid fist of the other. Let's get one thing straight…there is absolutely nothing fun about aspirations or biopsies or any other procedure requiring an eight-inch needle. Especially when the doctor comes in and says, "I can't aspirate these, they're solid. I'll just biopsy all three." Biopsies hurt. A lot. And you have absolutely zero opportunity to clench your teeth, or make a fist, or pound the table to help distract from the pain. When there's needle barreling its way through your boob, you take zero chances of moving. Instead, you cry silent, kind of whimper-y tears that aren't accompanied by any sound. You're barely getting enough oxygen to keep from passing out, holding your breath, hoping it will be over soon. It sounds like something out of Law & Order: SVU. (You just made the sound, didn't you? The #DoinkDoink…) And then it's over, the pain subsides, soreness and bruising sets in and you wait.

For those playing along at home, let's re-cap. In three weeks, I've had five doctors' appointments. Between the initial confirmation that I wasn't crazy, scans, bloodwork, and biopsies, I had been told probably in excess of 15 times that they were 'sure it was nothing.' I was 32, in relatively good health and had

ZERO family history of Breast Cancer. I didn't and still don't smoke (seriously, people – it's 2020!). I drank socially, had never done hard (read: any) drugs, didn't default to Styrofoam cups or food containers and didn't live near a power plant or power lines. Surely...*it was nothing.*

And then it was nothing. Radio silence for almost two weeks. All the anticipation, just to be left hanging. But what was I going to do? Dianne and I boarded the plane in Miami and went to Norway in search of the Northern Lights. Nothing like a 12-hour flight to sit and think about what the outcome could be. Nothing like a freezing cold destination to make you think about your boobs every time there was an icy breeze...Nothing like getting an email from your mom half way through Stockholm saying 'Your doctors called and want to make an appointment for when you're back.' Surely, *it was nothing.* I went online and made an appointment for the first week of February.

Our trip was fantastic. Aside from a few minor brushes with death thanks to a snow mobile and a wood-burning-stove-heated, clear-plexi-glass-roofed igloo inside the arctic circle, plus a lost wallet (#RookieMistake), we had an absolute blast. During our 10-day trip to Norway, Denmark and Sweden, we tried new foods and drinks, made invaluable memories, and eventually headed back to our normal lives in sunny south Florida.

Did I mention that throughout this whole story so far, I had been negotiating a brand-new job? Actually, *brand new* is probably the wrong term…I was being recruited over from the ad agency where I was an Account Director to work directly for my client, a sports broadcasting network, as a Strategist for the sales team. We were at the point where I had to make the agency aware of my intention to leave before the network would officially move forward with an offer. It was great timing. I was refreshed from my trip; my boss was about to leave on vacation, and I was giving plenty of notice. The offer wasn't official, and the entire conversation had been relatively theoretical up to this point. Monday and most of Tuesday were pretty much just two days of catch up after 10 days away. Tuesday afternoon, I went into the President's office and let him know that I was considering a job at the network and wanted to make him aware, especially due to the extremely close nature that we would continue to work together. He took it well, and I went home for the day, pumped and ready for whatever the future would hold. What a great way to end January!

Let's #RealTalk for a minute. You're a smart person. You knew when you picked up or ordered this book that it was about cancer; and I hope you've already deduced from the litany of tests I described what's coming next. But the purpose of this book is not to be some dramatic will-she/won't-she… I'm writing this #Cured, and I want you to know, #SpoilerAlert I'm fine.

However – you didn't stop watching Titanic after Jack was handcuffed to the boiler pipes (what a dick, by the way), so don't stop reading here. I promise, the read is worth it; but, sadly, and only because you asked, no; Leo does not

make a heroic cameo. Also, there was room on the door.

CHAPTER
THREE

FEBRUARY 1, 2017: D-DAY

I realize now that I had completely disregarded the fact that two separate doctors called my in-case-it's-serious-but-we-can't-get-ahold-of-you-contact while I was chasing the northern lights with Dianne. I'm not sure if deep down I knew it was bad news and was in denial, or if I really didn't expect anything to be wrong. I feel like cancer tests are something where you'd expect them to call you with the actual results either way – like a wedding RSVP or something – but it's still an enigma to me as to why I wasn't more worried about this appointment.

"I hate to be the bearer of bad news…" That's how she started immediately as she walked in the door of the exam room. No eye contact; surely, she was joking. That's the line I use when I'm 100% NOT about to tell someone something real, let alone something that will alter their anatomy. I partly expected the next words to be something like "You're not getting that boob job," or "You're not pregnant." We'd have a good laugh. I'd hug her for helping me through was could have been a horrible experience – thank God I was ok! – but that wasn't quite the message.

"The tests confirmed it. You have cancer."

I sat there, elbows on my knees, stunned. Shaking my head in disbelief, fidgeting with my cuticles.

She was fidget-y too. She had assured me – as had multiple others – that I had nothing to worry about. They were sure…WE were all so sure: *it was nothing*. We never even considered the alternate ending. We never planned how to deal with it or thought about the what-ifs; and we certainly didn't expect to even have to have 'the conversation.' She apologized – not like she did anything mal-practice-ish, but more like how you say you're sorry for someone's loss. She knew what was in store for me; how bad the diagnosis could actually be, and maybe a bit perturbed that she hadn't prepared me better for the news. Maybe I should have prepared myself…I don't know.

I couldn't look at her. I couldn't look at anything except my fidgeting fingers. As I blinked in rapid succession, water fell from my eyelashes to the floor. I couldn't think straight. I felt my entire world spin, my ears went into stereo, and all I could hear was white noise. You know in the movies, when someone is too close to an exploding bomb, so they get knocked 20-feet away, but they're alive and can't see straight or hear anything? But then the world slowly comes back into focus, and their senses return? The person who thought that up must have been served some pretty bad news at some point in their life, because that was me in the moments following the news. I took a deep breath.

"What do I – I don't even know what to…What's next?"

I have no idea what she said, but I left her office with a couple of phone numbers and some business cards.

I got into my car. I turned it on, put on my seatbelt and blasted the AC. And I completely lost my mind.

A little while ago – depending how fast you read – I took you through the five weeks of how I got to D-Day (Diagnosis Day). From the very beginning, through all the tests, I decided to play it close to the vest and keep it to myself, not telling anyone what was going on. Even as the tests got more specific, I wasn't convinced that anything would go unfavorably…It was no big deal and I was too young, with no family history. Plus, none of the seemingly hundreds of medical professionals I'd talked to seemed worried, so why should I be? It was my business, my health and my issue. But before I went on my trip, at the point that I still hadn't heard anything, I sat my parents down – just in case they got a call. Now, there's a bit of a backstory here.

Five years prior to my diagnosis, we lost my brother in a tragic motorcycle accident. My parents received a call from the police as they were driving home from a party. It was not good news, obviously, and to this day, any awkward-sounding start to a phone call freaks everyone out. I couldn't imagine them receiving a call to the tune of, "Hi, Mr./Mrs. Duemig? This is Doctor 'Smith' – Jessica put you as her emergency contact..." while I was 10,000 miles away, in the middle of the arctic circle with my sister. So, I sat them down prior to heading out of town.

I brought them up to speed about how I had found a lump, had been going through tests, and that I was sure it was nothing. 'But, in case you get a call while I'm away...yada, yada, yada.' They were alarmed, but I guess since I didn't seem worried, they weren't overly concerned. As I mentioned earlier, my mom let me know via email that she had received a call/the call, and basically, from that point on, it was a family affair. Both parents knew about my appointment on that day. They knew the time, and they knew that I likely wouldn't be in there for more than an hour.

So, sitting in my car, bawling by myself, freezing with the AC on, I called my mom.

"Hey Jess"

"Hi"

"Everything ok? How did it go?"

[Continue to lose my mind] "Um…not good."

"Why? What happened? You ok?"

"I…have…breast…cancer." [mind officially lost]

I don't really remember what happened next, other than that I cried and she cried a bit too. I think she asked me if I was able to drive. My dad called – beeped in on call waiting – and I told her that I couldn't tell him. She said she would do it for me (her first of many acts of sainthood) and we hung up; and I drove home. Barely.

I've since talked to my mom about this day and thanked her for how supportive she was. She remembers it well:

When Jessica first called me after her appointment and told me the diagnosis, I told her 'It's okay, everything will be fine, they'll do what they need to do; and you'll be done with it.' Then once it sunk in, and that it was both breasts, that it was a major surgery… I cried inside and out. But I needed to be strong for Jessica, be there for her to get through it. But inside I was dying. Was it my fault, did I pass on some cancer genes? I remember thinking those strands are so random. I even thought about how while I was pregnant with her, I worked with computers – could that have caused it?

By the time I got back to my apartment (about 10 minutes later), I had a text from my dad. He had talked to my mom and he didn't want to bug me; but he and my mom were there for me – for whatever I needed – and would be with me every step of the way. Whenever I was ready to talk, they'd be available. I had mentioned to my mom earlier that I didn't want anyone to know anything until I knew more, so they were sworn to secrecy.

I had every intention of laying in my bed, crying myself to sleep and figuring it all out tomorrow. But that was not how my afternoon went; after all, I was mid-negotiations on a new job. As they say in Miami, *no bueno*.

I called my dad, and he answered with a "That was quick." I told him I didn't want to talk about it – the infamous *it* – and that I had a bigger problem. I had to call my soon-to-be-new-boss and tell him the situation.

Okay, side note… Did I have to tell him? Probably not; but it's not in my nature to negotiate in bad faith; and having to take a significant amount of time off immediately after starting a new job – especially in a management position – is the definition of bad faith.

My dad assured me that this was the best way to go – honesty is the best policy – and that I probably didn't need any bad karma in my life right now. Also, in true dad form, he reasoned *if they wouldn't hire me because of this, did I really want to work for that company?* I thought through it a bit longer after I got off the phone with my dad and decided that I would tell my new boss about 'a medical issue' that had just come up. I cried some more…a medical issue. Wasn't that a bitch. UGHHHHHHHHHHHH.

I pulled myself together and made the call to my new boss. I gave him the news, a medical issue, and told him how it would require extremely quick action along with approximately six weeks of recovery. (By then some of the conversation I had had with the doctor was coming back to me.) I told him that I wanted to be upfront and that I would completely understand if the needs of the company were such that they required him to move in a different direction.

Without skipping a beat, he said, "Well, first of all, are you okay? [Yes, I will be.] Will this affect your head? (read: will you be brain-damaged? I think he was partially joking…) [Not in the long term.] Okay, well, I need to talk to some people here, but we want you on this team, and we've waited this long, so what's another couple of months? Let me make sure there's no issues and I'll get back to you." We hung up. I cried some more. I called my dad back. Told him about the conversation. And then at some point, I fell asleep.

The next morning sucked. Surprisingly I woke up on time, but my eyes were puffy, my body ached and I still couldn't eat. I showered and tried to figure out what to wear. Normally, I'd throw on some dress capris, a button down and flats, but today all I wanted was to wear something pretty. I've come to justify my actions as wanting to milk (pun intended) every last little bit of femininity out of the body that was betraying me. I'd soon undergo a massive surgery to remove both breasts and would never be the same again. So, joke's on you, cancer – I was going to wear a dress. A hot pink, form-fitting dress. And heels. Glorious heels.

I spoke with my parents again that morning and asked if they could send me flowers to work. I wanted to have something beautiful around me. I needed something sunny. They obliged, no questions asked. The questions came when I got a beautiful delivery of yellow roses... 'Oooooh!! Who's the guy?' Oh, girls, if only...

My 'new boss' called me early that afternoon and told me that the most important thing for me was to take care of whatever it was, that he was extremely impressed I thought it appropriate to give him the news, and that the network would be happy to have me as soon as I was ready. I was impressed that he was impressed. Did he expect anything less, especially given our four months conversations that had led to that point? Regardless, weight lifted. Well, weight #1.

Just two days prior, I had essentially given notice to the president of the ad agency that I was going to be applying for (he's not an idiot, most likely taking) the network job. Now I had to go back, tell him about my medical issue and explain my new timeline. I was paralyzed with the how, so I went to Human Resources for help. Luckily, the HR Director was an old family friend, someone that I had known seemingly forever, and the person who had recruited me into my current position. I told her the full story – about cancer, not a medical issue – and she talked me through the best way to communicate it to the President: she would do it for me. Later that day, The President called me into his office along with HR. He told me that I had his, their, the company's full support. That 'we were a family and we take care of our own. That this is why [I] have insurance; this is why [they] have insurance; and that [I] could do whatever [I] needed to do, take whatever time [I] needed to take for appointments, and just keep [them] posted regarding the bigger timeline – both of dealing with cancer, and leaving the agency.' I'm sorry, what?!

I was overcome. I thanked them and headed back to my office (seven feet away); and with about half a second to spare, I lost it…again. Weight #2, lifted.

CHAPTER
FOUR

GOOGLE

The next few days went by slow as molasses as I did everything I could not to Google anything. At this point, all I knew was that I had an official diagnosis of Triple Negative[3] breast cancer, and that I would see the Oncology Surgeon in the coming days to schedule surgery. Naturally, I did what any self-respecting honor student would do...I bought a binder. Yes, you read that right...a two-inch thick, hot pink (of course) binder that would come to be my medical Bible. It housed everything – paperwork, paperwork, paperwork...more paperwork. And receipts. So many receipts.

---

[3] Cancer.org, komen.org, and breastcancer.org have extensive information regarding receptor status of positive cancer pathology report

For the most part, I had decided to keep my diagnosis under wraps from the outside world until I knew more details about severity and treatment plan. I didn't want to raise alarm bells, and I also didn't want to downplay any of the details. The only people who were brought in on my secret were my grandparents and Godparents, and my parents, of course, who with my permission subsequently broke the news to my sister. They were all sworn to secrecy, except for talking to each other. I was getting pretty good at lying – or at least covering up my uncertainty and fear. It's funny how that works…I have cancer, I have the diagnosis, I have the long road ahead of me…and I'm the one consoling everyone else. I was surprisingly okay with this – I didn't need any more attention, and it was somehow cathartic to be strong. It seemed like the more I reassured everyone else that I was fine, that this was a minor speedbump and that cancer messed with the wrong girl, the more I actually believed it myself.

Telling my best friends was probably the hardest out of all the announcements. It's amazing how parents and grandparents are able to deal with news like this. They've seen a whole different world, for a whole lot longer. They've been through ordeals and situations that some of us will never even have to imagine…And they came through it, seemingly unscathed. They have a different perspective on life and health; and they're more equipped to deal with news of my sort.

Women my age…man, we are some fierce, strong, badass humans; but for the most part, we're not ready for news of this magnitude. My friends put on very strong faces – or ears, since it was over the phone – but I felt guilty telling them this news. They had their own lives, families, dogs, careers… But I needed them now and they knew it. And they were amazing. I never talked to them about how they took the news as it didn't seem like there was ever a right time to bring it up; and, quite frankly, I'm not sure I wanted to know.

I went about my business, trying desperately to avoid the occasional cry; and apparently did a pretty good job with it. My circle of trust was about 15 people strong and I could tell that not many other people were even suspicious that something was off. I was set to see the surgeon, so my parents came down to Miami to attend the appointment with me.

After the day I got diagnosed, I realized that the information that was to come in these appointments was extremely important, but also incredibly fleeting. In one ear and out the other – there's just too much to absorb, and too much to wrap your head around, too many big words. If you're reading this book because you've been recently diagnosed, it's super important that you either bring a voice recorder, a note pad or someone else with you to every single appointment.

Overall, I had been in better spirits, having come to terms with the reality of this life-changing news, but this is also when I learned maybe one of the most important lessons that would come from this whole ordeal:

Don't listen to people who have nothing constructive to say.

While I was busy avoiding Google, the few who knew about my predicament definitely were not; and suddenly I found myself surrounded by Internet MDs.

You probably won't need chemo.

Hey, here's a list of articles I found that talk about all the things you ate, drank or did to cause your cancer.

Ohh, triple negative…that's the easy one – you won't have to take the pill for the rest of your life! Win-win!

Jess – finally, the boob job you always wanted…

I can't lie, that last one was pretty funny (and I used it myself a time or two!). As much as I tried to take a step back and process everything on my own and prepare for the worst, I still wasn't ready for what the surgeon had to say.

She entered the exam room, introduced herself, shook our hands and sat down. The first thing out of her mouth once she sat down and we were ready to chat was… "Wow, that's a big binder." The look on her face said a lot more than that though. It said, "Shit. Here we go – another WebMD-er. I bet *she* is going to tell *me* all about her cancer…" I reassured her that this was just where I kept paperwork, notes and receipts and that I didn't know how else to organize it. She breathed. We laughed; and she told me 'Whatever [you] do, don't google anything.' Again, I reassured her and we were off to the races. Some people go through so many considerations in their own heads and from outside sources…Is this the right hospital? Should I get a second opinion? Should I have the surgery at all? Not me. Once the doctor came in, there was no question in my mind. My surgeon was an amazing woman – strong, stern, whip smart and no bullshit. Exactly the type of person I wanted to do my surgery.

"We're not going for treatment," she told me. "We're going for the cure."

That was reassuring. I like this chick!

"And then you'll do chemo."

Fuck.

This was definitely not the news I was expecting. Again, both the internet-certified doctors and some of the imaging techs along the way had weighed in on my condition and didn't expect that my specific case would require chemo. They were wrong (why did this surprise me?); and I was blindsided.

My parents were in the room with me when I got this news, but it's as if they weren't. I was in the middle of that mine field again. Stereo in my ears;

blinding white noise; head spinning. Suddenly I found myself unable to catch my breath. That was the day that the 500-pound gorilla sat on my chest.

My dad remembers it like it was yesterday:

The strength of my daughter, Jessica, is what helped me keep it together. I'm sure so many thoughts were swirling in her head, but her positive attitude and strength in the way she was handling it certainly had an effect on how I was getting through this. I remember when we first met with the surgeon and she gave Jess her diagnosis. It was so much more detailed and thorough than what her regular doctor had given. Rose [mom] and Jess were sitting up to the surgeon's desk and I was sitting behind them. I could see the giant tears (Jess always had giant tears) rolling down her face...then it seemed like she just shook them off, reset and took charge. At that point I knew she had this under control.

I regained my bearings, blinked the excess water from my eyes and breathed a very hollow, very releasing sigh. "I don't have time for this shit. What's the plan?"

The doctor walked me through what would become the immediate plan of action: a bi-lateral mastectomy with partial-reconstruction, including the removal of one or two lymph nodes for intraoperative testing with the possibility of removing them all in the event the cancer had infiltrated them. Shortly thereafter, I would undergo chemotherapy and possibly radiation before completing the reconstruction months later.

Partial Reconstruction happens during your first surgery. After the Oncology Surgeon is done removing all your breast tissue, the Plastic Surgeon inserts tissue expanders under your pectoral muscles. These tissue expanders each have a built-in port, which will allow the surgeon to add saline over the course of a few months. Adding saline increases the space, causing your muscles and skin to stretch, which prepares your body to accommodate permanent implants. Once it's safe to complete the reconstruction, usually after Chemo and Radiation, the Plastic Surgeon will remove the expanders and replace them with your permanent saline or silicone implants.

The Surgeon wanted to get in there and do the surgery as quickly as possibly due to the aggressive nature of Triple Negative Breast Cancer. The earliest she could get me into surgery was two and a half weeks away; and in the meantime, there was a laundry list of steps to complete. First, I had to schedule an appointment to see the Plastic Surgeon to get the 'before' photos and talk through my reconstructive options: things like implant material, shape, timing and general aesthetic goals. Then I would need to do a number of pre-operative tests and checks. I'd also need to see the Medical Oncologist to go through my chemo plans, as well as the Radiation Oncologist to determine whether or not radiation therapy would be required in addition to chemo. There was also genetic testing to be done – among everything else, BRCA1 and BRCA2.

I really don't know what happened the rest of that day. I'm pretty sure there was some crying. Mostly me, but also my mom and dad. It wasn't fair. I was only 32. No family history. No reason to even suspect the slightest possibility of a chance in a million that I would get this diagnosis. I didn't have time for it. I didn't have the patience for it. And I didn't want to deal with it.

I can't emphasize enough how great a role Miami Cancer Institute played in my overall experience with cancer. It was a one-stop-shop for all the cancer-specific facets of my treatment. While some of my appointments took place in South Miami (Plastic Surgery, Fertility Preservation), the majority of tests, doctors, surgeons, and other medical appointments were in one place. They shared a computer system, had centralized scheduling and even assigned me a "Nurse Navigator" to help me through the intricacies of my questions. If you are lucky enough to have the option of a single place for comprehensive care, I highly recommend factoring that into your overall decision-making process.

That weekend, during the short reprieve from a million and one tests, I went to the salon and cut my shoulder-length hair into a short pixie. Yay, control!

CHAPTER
FIVE

FEBRUARY 7TH. #SQUADGOALS

Once I had seemingly all of the pertinent information, I lifted the dome of secrecy from my parents and sister. We had to begin 'making arrangements,' as recovery time from surgery was to be at least two weeks. We debated whether or not it would make sense for me to stay with them about an hour and a half north, or some other plan, but once we realized the number of follow-up appointments I'd have to go to and factored in the distance from my house to MCI (a five-minute drive), it was clear: I'd stay at my own house.

I've already mentioned that my parents should be Canonized... but seriously, they were incredible. Thankfully, they both worked at very people-first companies, and my mom's boss allowed her to work from home (my home) for the two weeks following my surgery. The plan was that they would both come down from Wellington for the first surgery (a Friday) and stay through the weekend. On Sunday my dad would go home, and my mom would stay with me to help me maintain some semblance of self-sufficiency and take me to follow-up appointments.

The closer it got to surgery, the more time I had to be out of work. That, along with the constant puffiness in my face and the few times I forgot to take off my medical bracelet after appointments made it increasingly harder to keep the secret. I realized that this was pretty big news, and probably not something I would want to go through alone. Plus, I was eventually leaving my job – my staff would obviously find out, as would everyone else. So, I started telling people outside of the original few. It was very difficult and again I was in the position of reassuring everyone that I was going to be fine. But I soon realized that like that game of 'telephone' from childhood, misinformation was quickly spreading. All of a sudden, 'the cancer was stage four, and [I was] dying;' or 'a guy [I] was dating found the lump.' This was not going to work.

I thought about the best way to share my news and figured that Facebook would be an appropriate medium. I also realized that people are pretty sensitive on Facebook, and I wasn't planning to keep anything politically correct from that point on; so, I posted the following, public note:

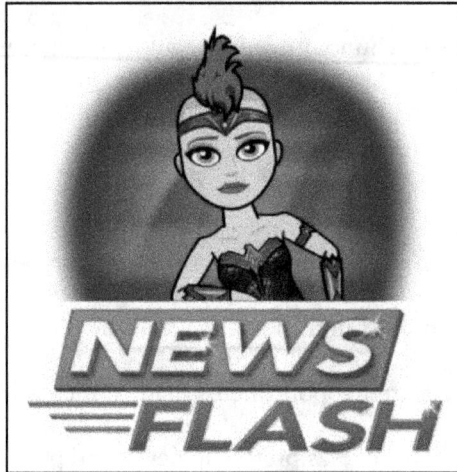

Hello friends and family! It's been a long time since I've been on Facebook; and it seems like every time I take a sabbatical, bad news brings me back. Unfortunately, this is one of those times. In a way, I'm thankful for this medium...it makes sharing news a bit easier.

That said, I wanted to share with you that I was recently diagnosed with stage 2 breast cancer. It's very aggressive and will be taken care of very quickly. I am in great spirits, ready for the challenge and anxious to kick ass.

The outpouring of support so far has been amazing and I'm so thankful – but it can definitely be a bit overwhelming. I know that people have different levels of acceptance on Facebook content, so I'm creating a group to keep those who want to be in the loop...in the loop ☺ It's a private, invite only group where I plan to share updates, so please let me know if you are interested in keeping up with what will be a challenging journey.

This doesn't mean I don't want and/or welcome phone calls, but I figure this will help with the dissemination of information.
Thanks for reading, and please comment below if you'd like to be added to the group!
XOXO

Honestly, I expected 25, maybe 30 people to opt-in to my group. I was beyond humbled when the group swelled to over 150 people, all offering their thoughts, prayers and good vibes. This group became exactly what I had hoped it would: a place for me to share important information, memes that made me laugh, uplifting stories and eventually, and maybe most importantly, live video updates. These videos would come to allow me to vent, to share my journey, and to have some sort of family/friend/human interaction as chemo progressed. Since I would be immunocompromised, I didn't plan to have guests over or really even leave the house myself in the beginning – with the exception of doctor visits, which were still plentiful.

A number of people in the group started asking me if they could invite someone they knew into the group because they were either going through the same thing I was, or had a family member who was, and they thought that person could benefit from hearing my story. After a short while, I decided to make the group public and allow anyone who wanted to join.

This group became my support squad, and the encouragement they shared with and for me was overwhelming at times. The good kind of overwhelming. In writing this book, I went back to that time capsule to re-read and re-watch the entire thread of the group[4]. WOW. I was – and continue to be – humbled.

---

[4] You can view my live videos at www.facebook.com/warriorguidebook, or at www.warriorguidebook.com

Sometimes, I can't believe that I made it through. Sometimes I don't recognize myself – who was that overly positive person who was speaking on those videos? Where did the logic and practicality come from? Where did the optimism and insight enter the picture? You know you had cancer, right? It's amazing what the mind can do when there's really only one thing to do: SURVIVE.

CHAPTER
SIX

SO MANY DECISIONS, SO LITTLE TIME

Twenty-one days: that's how much time I had from the day I received my diagnosis to the day the surgeon cut the cancer out of my chest. The countdown was on and the number of liters of blood taken from my arms was quickly rising. In just shy of three weeks, I had at least one doctor's appointment each day and bloodwork almost every day. Oncological Surgeon: Bloodwork. Radiation Oncologist: Bloodwork. Plastic Surgeon: Photos. Bloodwork. Genetic testing: Bloodwork. Surgical clearance: Echocardiogram[5]. Bloodwork.

---

[5] An Echocardiogram is an ultrasound of your heart. It's super cool and was a silver lining during this time!

I had to decide if I was on board with the double mastectomy, or if I wanted to go the single route. Did I want to get a second opinion? Did I want a port, which would protrude from my chest, have a tube directly into my heart and leave yet another scar, or did I prefer to do chemo through my regular veins and leave them collapsed, callused and rubbery? Credit or check? Did I want to see a psychologist before surgery? Did I want silicone or saline implants? Gummy bear or regular? Teardrop or round? What did I want to eat after surgery? Where was I going to live – my apartment or my parents' house? Which room in my house? Did I want to do fertility preservation? *Could* I do fertility preservation? Did I want to talk to others 'like me' who were going through this? Did I have a support group? I really should have a support group. Can we recommend a support group for you?

I think I made more decisions in those three weeks than I had in a collective very long time. What people on the outside sometimes don't realize is that all of these decisions on their own seem somewhat reasonable and like they should be relatively easy to make; but in my case, I was making them within days, even hours of one another. At some point, they all blend together. I recommend keeping a paper calendar.

Once I decided that my initial meeting with the Oncology Surgeon was enough to seal the deal, a second appointment was scheduled to walk through the surgery and plan all the details. One the day of the second appointment –

the Surgical Consult – I also met with a social worker and my Nurse Navigator. These two ladies were assigned to me to help me through the entire process over the months to follow, on everything from billing to where to go to buy a wig, to providing a list of people in my 'same shoes' that I could talk to. On this specific day, they also helped me with fertility preservation (freezing my eggs).

I had spoken with them briefly while I was in the waiting room to see my surgeon, and we broached the topic of fertility preservation. As I was heading to check out after the appointment, they pulled me aside and told me that given the date we had just scheduled surgery, and the plan to start chemo very quickly afterward, I had very little time to decide whether or not I wanted to harvest and freeze my eggs, let alone actually start the process. They told me that while I was in with the surgeon, they took the liberty of calling the fertility clinic, and the only opening they had for an initial consult was 'today at 11am.' It was 10:30 and we had to go straight there, right now. Otherwise, it wasn't going to happen. In just the two short weeks since diagnosis, my parents and I had realized that cancer appointments – and Miami traffic – are unpredictable, so we had adjusted our schedules to leave the afternoons open. In this scenario, it worked in my favor and off we went to South Miami for the fertility appointment.

It's also important to remember – whether it's you who is going through this, or if you're supporting someone who is – is that this rapid-fire decision making comes with the all-encompassing dark cloud of "This could kill me. I could literally die from the cancer, or from the surgery. It could turn out that none of these decisions even matter." Most of us never expected to have to deal with this or make any of the decisions that come with it. We've never questioned our mortality, or our self-worth, our legacy, or our femininity. We had plans. We had a fantastic life on the horizon and so many things we were supposed to do…and now we have to put that on hold – possibly indefinitely. I'm reminded of Mike Tyson's famous quote, "Everyone has a plan…until they get punched in the face." #IfEverThereWasAPunchToTheFace

When the surgeon talks about your surgery in broad terms like "bilateral mastectomy," she doesn't lead with the fact that she's going to cut clear across the middle of your breasts, take out all of your breast tissue – nipples included – and scrape your chest wall to ensure she gets all of it. She doesn't bullet-point that she's going to be literally an inch from your heart, lungs and several other vital organs. She'll mention drains, but not the details that she's going to be putting at least two puncture holes in each side of your torso, in the gaps between your ribs to make sure that the natural fluid accumulation can drain out of your chest cavity so that the trauma doesn't cause extra pressure on your lungs or heart. You'll have scars – big ones, and a lot of them, in lots of different places. You'll never be able to breastfeed your child – which you don't have yet, don't know if you ever even want, but could possibly never have now because chemotherapy could kill or damage every single one of your eggs (#FertilityPreservation). Things will look and feel different for both you and your significant other. You most likely won't even have nipples anymore – at least not as you've ever known them.

That Echocardiogram that they do during pre-op checks? That's to ensure that your heart pumps out at least 50% of the blood that's in there every time it contracts to make sure that not too much of the chemo drugs stay in the chamber, otherwise they could literally eat away at the muscle from the inside. The doctors and nurses have told you about every single complication that could happen with both surgery and chemo in a worst-case scenario setup. Don't eat this. Do eat that. Do you have a will? What about a living will? Don't go in the sun. Take Vitamin D pills. You look a little pale – are you going to pass out? Don't take too much medicine because it will constipate you. Take this medicine to get rid of the constipation. How do you feel? Do you feel lonely? Depressed? Do you feel like you still want to live? Have you had sad thoughts? On a scale on 1-10, how optimistic are you? (NOTE: These last few questions are very serious. Do not crack jokes. No one is amused, and you could be subjected to some legitimate counseling.)

Having to explain all this to your husband, your boyfriend, or some guy in the future, that you haven't met yet because you're single, is a battle in and of itself. How about every single person who asks you how you're feeling…?

What you think: [sarcasm] I'm great… except for, {VERBAL DIARRHEA}. Keeping my spirits up thanks to the Pinterest memes everyone keeps posting! Seriously? I have cancer and am in the hardest fight of my life – how do you think I'm feeling? Go fuck yourself.

What you say: Hangin' in there… One day at a time! 😊 (DEFLECT! DEFLECT! Quick, before you cry again!) How are you?

No matter what, you're likely going to second-guess every decision you make, and replay interpersonal communications over and over. (*Was I mean? Too mean?*) Unfortunately, that's just part of this whole ordeal. Let me reassure you of the power of your mindfulness…Though looking back it all feels like a blur, I think this 21-day period in the journey may have been the clearest my mind has ever been. I've heard that when you have to make a tough decision between two options, you should have someone simply flip a coin for you. Heads = option 1; tails = option 2. The point is not that you go with whichever option is associated with the side of the coin that lands face-up. In fact, you don't even have to (and probably shouldn't) look at it. The trick is that the second the coin is in the air, your mind will naturally hope for either heads or tails…That's your decision-maker. These 21 days between diagnosis and surgery were as clear as that coin flip. No time to think – only to decide. Like

Maverick said in *Top Gun,* "If you think, you're dead." A piece of advice: when in doubt, err on the conservative side – I may never use my frozen eggs, but at least I have the option.

CHAPTER
SEVEN

PREPARING FOR SURGERY: READ THIS IF YOU'RE THE PATIENT

irl, facing the idea of surgery is daunting and scary, but let's be real – these days, science is *so* advanced. Doctors are extremely qualified and as we've all seen on *Grey's Anatomy*, it's a cutthroat industry, where people fight and claw their ways to the top. To be the best. To be the most specialized. Their striving to be number one should be the most confidence-building part of this whole ordeal. Oncological Surgery – from what I am told and have experienced – is extremely difficult. So many things can go wrong and it's so meticulous that not just anyone can do it. Again – you will literally have the best of the best cutting open your chest.

The days after surgery will be tough. You'll come home wrapped tightly in ace bandages, with drains (you'll come to hate them in due time. Like five minutes.) pinned to your shirt. You'll likely be bloated and groggy and go right to sleep once you close the front door. Don't worry at all about sleeping the days away. Your body is working overtime to heal and get back to 'normal.' Listen to your body and let it do what it needs to do. Channel your inner Forrest Gump: when you're tired, sleep. When you're hungry, eat. When you're in pain, take a pill. There is no shame in any of that.

You will need help. From the day you're diagnosed, you'll need another set of ears, but after surgery, you'll need another set of hands too. Find someone – maybe a parent, a significant other, or a best friend – who is willing to help you with things you never thought you'd need. I know! You're strong, independent and self-sufficient. But you've never been through this before and there will be physical limitations that are 100% out of your control. Nobody is judging you for this, and needing help will actually prove to be more of a strength than a weakness in the long run. Be strong enough to ask for the help you know you need. Think about how you would react to a friend or family member in your shoes... You'd be there for them, no holds barred, right? Then let them help you. Now is not the time for pride – your journey will be hard enough.

Before surgery, you'll want to buy a number of front-fastening shirts. Whether they button down or snap closed, you won't be able to lift your arms over your head to put on a t-shirt. You'll go from hot to cold quickly too, so mix it up with long- and short-sleeve options. Find a zippered hoodie as well. There's one very serious thing you should know about this part... I'm sorry to have to be the one to tell you this, but you may end up looking like a lumberjack. Depending on the time of the year of your surgery, loose-fitting button downs may be hard to come by. But you're in luck! You know what never seems to go out of style? Flannel. Pick your color and wear it like a champ. (Disclaimer: don't try to chop wood.)

Before you go in for your surgery, be sure to shave your legs and underarms (if this is part of your normal routine), because showering on your own will be extremely difficult and shaving will be the last thing you want to deal with. Could be a while before that is re-prioritized. But remember! The doctors are going to ask you to shower with a special anti-microbial soap the night before and the morning of your surgery. Shave your legs the day before you have to use that soap, otherwise it will burn. (It's the little things, people!)

Make sure you have an alternative sleeping spot set up before you go to the hospital for your surgery. A recliner is great, but even something as simple as a lower-to-the-ground mattress can make a world of difference.

To set the scene, at the time of my surgery, I lived alone in a high rise in South Miami. I had 14-foot ceilings, and an open floor plan. My bed put my mattress about 36 inches off the ground, my kitchen cabinets were extra tall, given the height of the ceilings and I had a stacked washer and dryer. For many days after surgery, I wasn't able to move my arms above parallel to the floor, so it is extremely important to understand the impending restrictions and get your dwelling set up ahead of your surgery day. Suddenly things like getting a glass from the cabinet or ice water from the fridge were impossible. Whether from warnings or fear of the unknown, my entire body, from the waist up, moved as one rigid piece. When you've been restricted to a hospital bed for two days, the thing you want most – aside from food – is to sleep in your own bed. Put this book down and go get into your bed. Snuggle up and get comfortable. Hell, take a nap! I'll wait.

* * *

How was it? Did you untuck the top sheet and peel it back with the comforter? Put both hands on the bed for support and raise your knee to ultimately tumble into the softness? Did you lay on your back, palms down and brace yourself to scoot your butt into the perfect spot, use your abs to lower your head to the pillow and back up to reach for the covers, only to flip onto your side? Are you a stomach sleeper?

All of these actions will be all but impossible in your first few days home, but you'll figure out the best tips and tricks that work for you as you get comfortable with your pain tolerance and as you overcome the initial fears of what your body can and can't do. I slept at a 45-degree angle, created by multiple pillows. I slept in the middle of the bed so that I could have pillows on either side of me to rest my arms in a comfortable position. You may want to get a travel neck pillow to keep your head from jerking around throughout the night but you may want to try sleeping without it at first. Eventually you'll get more and more comfortable and the anxiety of going to bed will subside. Just be prepared for things to be difficult for a while – especially while you have the drains. Normally, I am a side sleeper, so as I got comfortable easing over by about five degrees night by night, I found that placing a pair of socks between my boobs helped with comfort and support. If you remember, my tissue expanders were only about 150-200ccs total, so there wasn't much actual 'boob' to support. It's hard to explain, but because you'll likely have very little (if any) feeling in your chest, nerves that are active will be in hyperdrive. I found that this made my chest felt extremely heavy, both when I was on my back and when I was on my side, so even the smallest bit of support seemed to do wonders and put my mind at ease enough to doze off.

As for navigating your kitchen and day-to-day tasks, you really will need help here. For the first few days, someone else will need to do the little things for you. Of course, try to do as much house cleaning (laundry, dishes, maybe even meal prep) before you even go into surgery, but also recognize that none of that stuff will even matter when you're sitting around in elastic-banded pants and button-down shirts once you're home. You'll hardly need dishes for the food you won't really be in the mood to eat, and your best bet is probably going to be to get some sort of cold-preserving cup to use over and over – maybe a YETI or Tervis Tumbler. Grab some paper plates, napkins or paper towels and set them out on the counter, next to where you'll place your medications and prescriptions. Your setup may seem disheveled and overwhelming, but it's not the end of the world. As your bandages come off, and you start getting back to a normal-ish routine, remember that you will have very little upper body strength, so lifting even something like a pot to the stove could be difficult! You'll be surprised to feel just how engaged your pectoral muscles are in everyday tasks.

You won't be able to shower for the first couple of days after you come home from the hospital. I found baby wipes to be very helpful during this time. They will keep you clean in all the right areas and will help deter any body odor. Luckily you won't be too active, so you'll be fine in regards to sweat; but your body will be dispelling excess hydration and drugs from the surgery, so while you may not feel particularly 'dirty,' it's important to get those substances off your skin. Once you are able to shower – both from the Doctor's perspective and your own level of comfort – beware that hot may feel hotter and cold may feel colder than usual. You will need help showering. You're going to feel very weird asking someone to help you wash your hair, but you have to. You won't physically be able to do it yourself at first, so just suck it up. By now, your helper has emptied your drains, so their *ew* level has a really high bar. Of all the things to come for you, this should not be something you think twice about. Plus, who doesn't love a scalp massage? By the way, aren't you glad you shaved your legs?

You need to allow yourself to cry. I read somewhere about tribes of people in other parts of the world that experience loss in a much different way than we're conditioned to do so in our feelings-are-bad society. When one of these people – mostly women in this case – lose someone, they go away from the village and wail for as long as it takes. They scream and cry and moan toward the forest or the ocean and literally expel the stress, anxiety and emotion out of their bodies forever.

The shower was my beach, my forest, my crying place. It was the only place (after the first few post-surgery trips) that I was truly alone and had zero distractions. It was where I could think and react and breakdown without anyone knowing, or asking me what was wrong, or consoling me. Sometimes I would sit on the floor of the tub just letting the water cascade over me; other times, I placed my hands on the wall with my head down or faced the water stream directly. No matter the position, this was an essential part of my healing because sometimes, you really just need to get it out. Tears are cleansing – they cleanse our minds and our souls.

As much as you are hurting, and as angry as you may be, always remember that this is also affecting your loved ones and those who love you equally, if not more. For example, my dad had a really hard time with not being able to fix my situation:

The hardest part for me personally was not being able to "fix it!" I'm the dad...I am supposed to be the guy who fixes everything for the kids. Before all this, I was able to fix everything: make the kids' lives easier, teach them different lifelong lessons, give them great, and I mean great, words to live by like "Quitters never win and winners never quit!" Jess was obviously a winner, so it was a feeling of uselessness. What good am I if I can't fix this? What's the right thing to say that will fix it? What's the right thing to do to fix it? Watching a daughter I love so much enduring such a difficult time in her life, and not being able to fix it? That was the worst.

My mom also had similar feelings:

The hardest part for me was that my baby was hurt, and I couldn't do anything to make it go away. When she was little and had a cold, I could help her by putting a little Vicks (VapoRub) on her chest. Some medicine and hugs, and she would be okay. This was out of my hands... I just wanted to hold her and hide her from it all. But she was stronger than I expected. She shook it off and took control of as much of it as she could. I made sure I was there for her when she wanted me to be there, as much as she needed me to be there. And then I cried some more.

Make sure you count your blessings and acknowledge and thank those who are helping you. Even a simple check-in from someone, be it a Facebook comment or text message, can change your entire outlook for the day. It could give you the little bit of a recharge that you didn't even know you needed. If you find yourself in a position where you feel like you don't have anyone who can help you, there are definitely resources at your hospital or cancer center. If all else fails, join my Facebook group and you'll have the power of the community behind you!

CHAPTER
EIGHT

PREPARING FOR SURGERY: READ THIS IF YOU'RE A SUPPORTER

I'm going to talk to the supporters here for a minute. If you're one of the amazing people who will be helping someone through the hardest, scariest fight of their life – for their life – kudos. You are a kind soul who likely has a spot reserved for you in Heaven. I know you're not the one fighting, but this is going to be a difficult journey for you as well. But I want to help you understand the what, why and how, because the person you're taking care of will never tell you.

When they first receive the diagnosis, it won't sink in right away. There will be the initial emotional response, but then there will be a very weird "Fuck this shit" attitude that sets in. It could be one of denial or of stepping up to the challenge that awaits them. Try to identify early which way they're swaying, although it could change a few times in the initial eight hours, until they go to bed or take a shower...whichever comes first. Then will come the tears. The mental anguish of 'this isn't happening, let alone to me.' Then the over-analysis: What did I do to deserve this? What did I eat? Smoke? Wear? Drink? Breathe? Did getting hit in the chest with a soccer ball for 12 years cause this? Was it my bra? Should I have skipped the underwire? Should I not have worn a sports bra so much? Did I need more support? Less? Was it my sex life? Was it environmental? Power lines? Lead in the water? Cell phone use? ...And that's just day one.

Days two through seven-ish will be a blur for everyone involved as surgeries are scheduled, pre-op appointments are made, they're detoxing from ibuprofen and aspirin and winding down projects at work and home. Please don't forget that any time the patient is alone and/or not distracted, they will go to the darkest place in their mind. They will see cancer everywhere. They will see death everywhere. They will question every possible outcome in a downward spiral of what if? The fear of the unknown will take over and be all-encompassing.

Facing the idea of surgery is daunting and scary. So many things can go wrong, but Oncological Surgery is so meticulous and so difficult to master that not just any surgeon can step in and do it. Years of training and practice and mastery has gone into their surgeon picking up that scalpel. Help the patient understand that while worrying won't help anything, they're in great hands nonetheless. Sometimes, all they will need is a strong embrace and to know that you're there for them.

If you're a parent to the patient, know that having you there to help them through this is the best and worst feeling of their lives. Chances are your patient is strong and independent, self-sufficient and proud. She's also scared and a bit ashamed. I know! It doesn't make sense... She did nothing to bring this on herself, and there's nothing she could have done differently to stop it, but she still feels beside herself that she needs anyone, let alone her parents. She's also extremely grateful that you're there.

If you're a significant other to the patient, see above. But there's also a whole other level to this when it comes to you. As far as she's concerned, she's about to be mangled. I know! It could not possibly be that bad...but to her, anything less than the original recipe will likely make her feel this way. I had two phenomenal surgeons. My Oncology Surgeon – the one who took everything out – was thorough and efficient. She managed to keep the incisions as small as possible, but they were still about eight inches long and half an inch thick by the time they fully healed. My Plastic Surgeon – the one who put everything in – was fantastic as well. He kept the scars as thin and clean as possible, and the placement of my implants is so natural looking that people sometimes don't believe I had a double mastectomy. It doesn't matter. Her breasts are not the way they were: the scars are there, and no matter how much they may or may not fade, she won't want anyone to see them. Oh yeah – she may lose her nipples. (That part will depend on the type of cancer the patient has, and the surgical plan.) The bottom line is that there will be adjustments – things will feel different for you, and they'll feel different for her (if she can feel anything at all). You need to decide very early on whether or not you want to be along for the roller coaster ride. If you're in, be all-in. If you're out, get the fuck out, preferably sooner rather than later.

A special note for the dads out there. Your daughter's breasts are no longer breasts. They might as well be her big toe. (There's a visual!) She won't see them as sexual or private and neither should you. If you are in the position where you're her sole caretaker, just go with it, but have an honest, open conversation early on about insecurities, boundaries and logistics if you feel it will help. My dad was not my sole caretaker, and I didn't need him to help with some of the more sensitive or intimate tasks. After it was all over, he shared with me what he would change if he had to (God forbid) go back and do it all over again:

Of course, the first thing I would change is the diagnosis. I guess I would have liked to spend more time with Jess as she was going through this. Maybe visiting her more and planning some fun things to do. I think her surgeons and doctors were great and the treatment at the hospitals were excellent.

Everything went as well as we could have imagined. But maybe I could have made some plans to do some fun stuff and visited more often. Maybe I could have sent more flowers or mailed her a gift for no reason.

The days after surgery will be tough for the patient and relatively easy – albeit boring – for you. She'll come home wrapped tightly in ace bandages, with drains pinned to her shirt. The drains will be the worst part – for both of you. They'll constantly be in her way and you'll be the one cleaning these out for the first few days. (I would highly recommend watching very gory movies to prepare. Don't look at me that way – it's gross.) She'll sleep a lot – mostly because of the pain medication, but also because her body is, you know, recovering from major surgery. Let her sleep. Her body will be extremely sensitive coming off of the anesthesia and there will be a number of things she won't be able to do for herself the first few days, so be supportive and touch her with kid gloves. After a couple of days of fear of the unknown, she'll realize she doesn't actually need the pain medication much anymore and will likely wean herself off. She'll start to do things for herself and will push the boundaries. Let her push them. Trust me, she'll ask you for help when she needs it.

One thing to be aware of is that surgery wreaks havoc on the digestive system. Between the very little bit she'll be eating and the propensity for the medications to mess with her stomach, she may become constipated without realizing it. She'll likely lose track of her bowel movements amidst her random sleep and medication schedule (if you can call it a schedule), and this can become a troublesome situation. I recommend being prepared with a laxative just in case.

She should have bought a number of front-fastening shirts ahead of time. Whether they button down or snap closed, they're going to make her want to punch a wall. All of the emotions she's carrying will manifest themselves in that God-damn 3rd button, and there may be a meltdown. Prepare yourself, let it happen and offer to help. Don't be surprised if she snaps at you and wants to fight with it herself. She'll get there.

She won't shower for the first few days. I found baby wipes to come in very handy during this time. Obviously, you will need to wait for the doctors to green light her showering privileges, but even then she may be a bit reluctant. Remember, she already feels 10 times more gross than you think she smells, but she's probably never had her chest cut open before and doesn't know what to expect; so be nice, but also, nudge her. She will thank you later. The first time in the shower could be tough. Surgery changes things and your sensations could be elevated. Hot will be hotter. Cold will be colder. Be careful with that first shower.

Also, the fucking drains. Technically, they're attached to her skin at the entry point with a single stitch; but they'll be heavy and will feel like they're pulling out of her ribs, especially when carrying the weight of a water stream.

They're not pulling out of her – wait until you see them actually being taken out. The best bet is to empty them before the shower, and then create a device to hang them while in the shower. I used a simple white rope – something my dad brought from his garage – and looped it around my neck. As I got more comfortable (read: over it), I used a plastic clothes hanger to secure them away from me and onto the shower curtain bar. Game changer.

Finally, remember she won't be able to lift her arms above parallel to the floor. Part of this is because of doctors' orders, part is because of the fear of the unknown. Either way, she'll need help washing her hair. It's awkward, you'll likely get soaked, and you'll both end up laughing then crying, but this is something she'll remember as endearing and will love you more for helping her secure this small part of normal.

I was at my lowest, darkest points in the shower. It was the only place (after the first few post-surgery trips that my mom helped me with) that I was truly alone and had zero distractions. It was where I could think and react and breakdown without anyone knowing, or asking me what was wrong, or consoling me. Sometimes, she just needs to cry it out.

My parents were my biggest cheerleaders and my greatest support during my journey. I asked them to provide some advice for those of you to whom this chapter especially pertains:

There is no right way to help your loved one - just be there and take your cue from them. Obviously with a small child, you have more control, but you're also needed so much more. With an older person, whether it be a parent, sibling, child or otherwise, just be there for them when they need you, to listen, to help care for them, to be their sounding board and their shoulder to cry on. Hug them, laugh with them, be positive for them and most of all let them know you love them beyond infinity and back.

Be present and positive. Listen sometimes and don't try to "fix it." Go to doctors' appointments but don't be hurt if they want to go alone. Most importantly, if you believe, pray and keep the faith. Be positive and maybe reach out to other parents that have experienced similar experiences. Knowing you aren't alone in this is critical. That can give you an outlet that you may not want your child or loved one to have to hear. If you are married, lean on one another. This is critical because at different times one of you will be stronger than the other. So being able to talk to each other and lean on each other is so important. I believe with both of our experiences (with Jimmy then Jess), our marriage grew stronger and my relationship with my wife became closer. Sometimes, even now, we know without saying anything, that one of us are going through a tough time thinking about our kids... So be there for your loved one, listen to them, pray, reach out to others and let others reach out to you.

CHAPTER
NINE

SURGERY

Out of nowhere, it was the 22nd and I was up early and over to the hospital, where I was taken to surgical prep pretty quickly. I was almost ready to go into the operating room, but before we could get the show on the road, I needed to have my IV placed. The nurse, who was very obviously and very hysterically the jokester of the group, took my left hand, which had the better, juicier vein, and as he inserted the needle, popped it like a water balloon. My hand was instantly full of blood, so much so that it dripped on the floor. (Tourniquets work!) He apologized, noting that this wasn't an uncommon occurrence, and nonchalantly wiped off my hand. No big deal. You should have seen the surgeon's face when she walked into my curtained off bay in the surgery preparation area.

With half a chuckle at what was an extremely overdramatic looking scenario, she blurted out, "What the heck happened here?!" I told her the story and she did one of those faces that said, 'sounds about right.' "But why did they put it in your left arm?" I looked at her with a blank, you're-the-doctor stare. (I came to realize that the reason she didn't want the IV in my left arm was because that was the side with the cancer, and during surgery, she'd need access to my left arm pit to access, excise and test my lymph nodes. Not an easy task when the patient's hand is tethered to an IV drip.) "It doesn't matter, we'll switch it once you're out (read: unconscious)." And then I was out.

From an outsider's perspective, you could be reading this and thinking, "What the fuck? How are they laughing about this situation? And how is she so okay with them putting the IV in the wrong arm?" But you have to take the levity where you can in situations as grave as a cancer diagnosis. February and March are very difficult months for my family. In 2012, we lost my brother in a motorcycle accident at the end of March, just a month and change after his 24th birthday on February 21st. I'm sure you can imagine the challenge of getting a cancer diagnosis, and subsequent surgery date within the same month, followed by a chemo start date of just weeks later. It was mental, emotional, psychological, physical... overload. Little moments like this, where we could all laugh in the face of a major surgery, were important and kind of a blessing.

I don't remember much of the rest of that day, but I do know that surgery was only supposed to take a few hours. Ha – 'only.' So it was a chaotic scene when they rolled me into my room at close to 11pm. Despite coming off of some pretty heavy anesthesia, I was able to calculate that 11pm was much later than I should have returned, and in my woozy, half-lucid state, I was convinced that something had gone terribly wrong. Had I experienced some sort of complication on the table? Were they able to complete the surgery as planned? Did I die? What the hell was going on? Why was it almost 12 hours later? I was freaking out and it was not a good feeling. But my parents were there in the room when they rolled me in, and ultimately, I was fine. As it turned out, all the hoopla around the time lapse between when I was taken into surgery and when I came out was for naught. Due to a bit of overcrowding or poor planning – I didn't ask – the hospital had to wait for an open room before locking me in for the night, so they simply kept me in recovery longer than usual.

The next few days are fuzzy. It's such a weird feeling, not remembering. Maybe it's a self-preservation instinct; or maybe a psychiatric phenomenon. Maybe it's just sheer mental overload… but it's very unsettling. I see pictures (Oh God, the pictures!) and I think I remember being in that place at that time, but I can't honestly say I remember being in that moment. I think to myself, "First my body turns on me; now my mind…What's next?!" Somehow, on February 23rd, I returned home – my money is on my parents driving me

– and there I slept. I think.

CHAPTER
TEN

SETTLING IN AND NEXT STEPS

I t feels weird to say it now, but surgery was kind of the easy part. There were really no questions to be answered regarding that part of the process. Double mastectomy: check. Partial reconstruction: check. Chemo port: check. Drains (fucking drains): check. The word 'auto-pilot' comes to mind.

Even the first couple of days – or was it hours – of recovery itself weren't too bad. When I was awake, I was uncomfortable and groggy from the pain medication, so the majority of my time was spent watching mindless television or sleeping. For the first time in three weeks, I had nothing to think about except the backs of my eyelids. I rested. My mind was at peace – if for no other reason than the Percocet. Take it where you can get it, girls!

One morning, I woke up in a particularly chipper mood, which was quite possibly a lingering effect of the Percocet from the night before. I had fashioned a temporary holder for my drains using the belt of an old bath robe, two drains tied to each end, resting over my shoulders, both ends in the front. I was in stitches because the belt, held taught by the weight of the drain bulbs hung even with my hips. I ran out of my room and startled my mom who was sitting at her computer on the couch, as I yelled, "They gave me the wrong surgery! I have BALLS!!! FOUR BALLS!!!" If I hadn't just had surgery, I probably would have been rolling on the floor. I don't think I was actually high, but I cracked myself up and, in that moment, that's all that mattered.

Aside from my couch naps, overnight sleeping was pretty unbearable. Between taking residence in the guest room since my bed was too high to even get into, being warm and unable to cool off at all times and having to sleep sitting up, I was miserable and spent most nights silently crying myself to sleep. The drains were already taking their toll on me. I couldn't navigate them. The tubes from my ribs to the fluid-filled balls at the ends were twisty and awkward. They always seemed to be in the way, and I was constantly worried about them opening up and leaking all over everything. It seems so insignificant and so trivial but recovering was like death by 1,000 cuts. Remember you're talking to the girl who moved out of a great apartment in Tampa solely because of the ridiculous height of the speed bumps in the neighborhood. My only defense to that is thank God I didn't live in that neighborhood during this!

We were finally able to get into a routine and I found a comfortable sleeping position. I even devised a contraption to house the drains, thanks to four can koozies and an old belt. All was well for the moment.

After surgery, once you wean yourself off the pain pills, your body feels very strange – like it's not there. Oddly enough, it is 'not there,' and what's left 'there' is a whole lot of nerve damage. I think the pain pills are prescribed more for their put-you-to-sleep powers, rather than the dulling-the-pain powers. With all the tissue that was removed, the nerves are barely intact, if at all – I didn't feel anything. Good or bad. Sometimes I wanted to feel something to make sure the whole thing was real and not a bad nightmare, but the minute I received some sort of twinge from a remnant nerve ending, I regretted the request to my body and started to settle for nada.

Even now, as I close my eyes and move my index finger across or around my chest, there are very distinct boundaries to the numbness; and pressure replaces any sort of actual, tangible feeling. I can feel adjacent to the surgical field, but where I should have felt nipple constriction (like when you're cold) or muscles flexing, I experience the feeling you get when you sit for too long and your foot falls asleep, but you still need to walk somewhere. You know the foot is there, it's sturdy and you have some control over it, but you can't expressly feel it. But this is on your chest... It's a very weird phenomenon!

After you've had your breasts removed, it seems a bit redundant to wear a bra, but at the beginning, the bra was essential for keeping the bandages in place. The bra they sent me home from the hospital in was made from a very thin material, had a couple of seams and clasped in the front. It was also itchy, could never get situated correctly, seemed to make the pressure worse and was extremely warm. Even despite a 74-degree apartment, anytime I was wearing that bra, I was sweating. In hindsight, it might have been the fertility shots and subsequent perimenopause, or maybe just anxiety from the whole situation.

Whenever I needed a break from the heat and itchiness, I would simply take it off and walk around the house topless. It was just me and my mom by this point, so it was no big deal. I say it was nothing my mom hadn't seen before, but my chest was far from natural looking. As painful as it was for her to see my scarred chest, she never mentioned it or made me feel awkward (#Saint). The concept of walking around without a shirt on was super weird because I had never done it before, but it was so comfortable. Man! Guys have it made! On days like that, I would just sit in the chair, under the AC vent, with my feet up, steadied by pillows, hands folded on my stomach and breathe. I usually fell asleep in this position and those were some of the soundest hours of sleep I got for a long time.

In the first few days after I came home from the hospital after my mastectomy, I had multiple follow ups with both surgeons, as well as consultations and education sessions with the Medical Oncologist and the Chemotherapy Education team. We outlined my regimen, decided on frequency, and scheduled the appointments. My plastic surgeon inflated my tissue expanders as much as possible in the weeks between surgery and chemo because once chemo started, the risk of infection was too high.

In that time, I also spoke to two Radiation Oncologists (both USF grads, #GoBulls) and we agreed that radiation could not guarantee anything, so I decided to forego this part of treatment. Just to triple check, I asked the doctors, "If I told you right now, I'm not going to take radiation and walked out of the room, would you chase me and try to convince me otherwise? Are the statistics that much in favor that I'd be an idiot not to do it?" They answered honestly and it was decided. No radiation.

I had seen a fertility specialist the week before my surgery. We discussed my diagnosis and the potential outcome of chemotherapy. There was a pretty decent chance, given my age, that chemo would wipe out or at least render damaged the remainder of my eggs, and that I would likely have a hard time conceiving a child naturally.

That was pretty tough to hear, but my reaction to it was also quite unexpected. I had never been hell-bent on becoming a mom. I thought I had made the decision to remain childless for life years prior as I was building my career. Or maybe that's just what I told myself to stave off unwanted pregnancy – I'm not really sure anymore. I realized that it's very easy to *decide* what you do or don't want when you have the safety net of being able to change your mind. But suddenly they were telling me I might not be able to have kids at all, essentially removing that safety net. What was already a no-brainer for me became a very different no-brainer: I decided that the best plan was to harvest and freeze my eggs.

This process isn't for the faint of heart. No matter how comfortable I got (are you ever really comfortable?) with needles and being poked and prodded, nothing prepares you to do it to yourself. There are literally instincts in your brain whose only jobs are to prevent you from hurting yourself. The first step in the process of egg harvesting entails self-administering hormones[6] (via syringe). These hormones stimulate your ovaries to mass-produce follicles, which is where the eggs live within your ovaries. Each egg gets its own follicle. During a normal menstrual cycle, you have one, maybe two follicles doing their thing. These drugs spark four to 10 follicles into action! As I'm sure you can

---

[6] If you are considering fertility preservation, be sure to ask your health professionals about benefits from LiveStrong and Walgreens. As long as you meet certain income thresholds, there is financial aid for cancer patients as it applies to fertility and it can significantly reduce some of the stressors.

imagine, this also stimulates the equivalent of PMS times ten (#MySaintlyParents).

Once your follicles and respective eggs mature, another drug – also self-injected – referred to as 'the trigger shot' causes the eggs to ovulate, or release, from the follicles into the fallopian tubes. Once this takes place, the doctor goes into the fallopian tubes – there's really only one way to get there, use your imagination – and retrieves the eggs with a needle. The whole process is extremely regimented with specific doses on specific days, and intravaginal ultrasounds to ensure maturity. Doing it incorrectly can result in fewer or unusable, immature eggs. Also, there is nothing mature about cracking sex toy jokes in the middle of an appointment. #LessonLearned #TheyveHeardItAll

I couldn't start this regimen prior to surgery since the hormones could interfere with the process and plan, and I certainly couldn't start it once chemo commenced and mix everything together. I also had to do more tests to make sure my body was ready for chemo, so I had less than 16 days to complete what in normal cases of Invitro Fertilization would be a four- to six-week process. After completing mounds of paperwork, and accounting for the transfer of my frozen eggs for every situation under the sun that I may or may not encounter over the next 60 years of my life, I started the shots the day I returned home from the hospital. Eight days later, I had four viable eggs retrieved.

Those were very long days. I had five doctor's appointments in eight days – sometimes multiples in the same day. It was tiring, it was draining (literally – most days included blood draws!), and it was expensive. My eggs are now frozen safely somewhere in Central Florida. I like to think they're parked somewhere between Walt Disney and Austin Powers! To this day, I'm still not sure that I will use my 'oocytes' as they're called, but at least I have the option.

CHAPTER
ELEVEN

CHEMOTHERAPY

This chapter will be a tough one – to write and to read – but I want you to know what you're getting into here – and I want you to hear it from me. Not that you have much of a choice when it comes to whether or not you'll indeed have to endure chemo, but I want you to hear this from a real person who experienced it – not someone who is covering their ass at the hospital. The nurses and doctors are fantastic, but they're going to walk you through the absolute worst-case scenarios, every side effect under the sun and make you think you're going to die. They're going to caveat the treatment until they're blue in the face and make you prepare for things that may not ever happen to you. You'll spend so much money on stuff you may never need, and you'll go into each treatment thinking it may be your last.

Full transparency: it might be. You could die. You could also get hit by a bus on your way to McDonald's. Or you could die peacefully in your sleep in 60 years, having lived a full, enriched, silicone-breasted life. You CANNOT live your life in fear. Not in fear of cancer. Not in fear of chemo. Not in fear of recovery. Not in fear of the unknown. I hope that reading this chapter and the next will take away your fear, add some levity and ultimately make at least some of the journey known. In a perfect world, you'll inherit my #FuckCancer attitude, take pity on those cancer cells for having picked the wrong body to inhabit and never look back. Either way, find your strength in whatever form it comes, and milk it for all you can when you find it because it will come and go. Some days you will feel strong and on top of the world. Other days, you'll curl up in a ball on the couch and cry. You'll be tired and cranky and happy and elated and depressed and itchy and hot and cold. But you'll be strong. And I'm confident you'll come out victorious.

Do you know how chemotherapy works? Chemo – we're on a nick name basis – is basically acid disguised as medicine that attacks the fast-splitting/growing/multiplying cells in your body: cancer cells – obviously that's why it works; taste buds – why some people get weird metal tastes or lose their desire for certain foods/drinks; hair follicles – why some people lose their hair; and reproductive cells (your eggs) – why some people are never able to have children afterward.

I was officially diagnosed Stage 2A, which meant my cancer was between two and five centimeters (the size of a lime) and had not spread to the lymph nodes under my left arm. Why is lymph node involvement important? For those of you who were not science majors, lymph nodes are part of the immune system and exist to filter your blood from all harmful substances. They also help with absorption of fatty acids, but in short, all of your blood passes through these *filters*. Imagine using a coffee filter a second day in a row – or worse, with a few days in between… The remnant coffee grinds will affect the new water passing through and could potentially sour the new pot of liquid gold. Similar situation here, where all of the blood that passes through the lymph nodes could have served as trollies, transporting the cancer cells to other parts of my body.

Thanks to the timing between when I found the lump in my left breast, the tests, the plan, and surgery, I was very lucky that the cancer hadn't spread to my lymph nodes. However, despite the radically conservative mastectomy where my surgeon was able to achieve clean margins, Chemo was required to ensure that none of those little bastards (read: cancer cells) escaped. I would be required to do eight rounds of chemotherapy (four treatments of one type, then four treatments of another) over the months to follow. The plan was to test out doing a treatment every two weeks, but more likely, it would be stretched to every three weeks to allow my body additional time to recover between treatments.

Chemo is a very grueling process. Not the treatments themselves – basically you're just sitting in a recliner for a few hours – but the rigamarole that happens in between. In general – and remember everyone's regimens are different – here's what you can expect:

The morning of chemo, you go in early for blood tests to get a count of your white blood cells. They must be at a certain threshold because the chemo is going to wipe them out, and obviously they can't actually be at zero. So, assuming they're high enough, you'll go in and sit for somewhere around five hours for the chemo treatment itself. The next day, although it seems the technology has changed a bit since I had my treatments, you'll have more blood work (your white blood cells will have tanked by now), and get a shot of more medicine (Neulasta, ~$8k per shot) that will help your white blood cells regenerate. If your counts are too low, they will have to give you antibiotics to help protect against infection. Then you will feel like garbage for a week before going back and doing it all over again, for as many rounds as are required. It's tiring and nerve-wracking. Your immune system is compromised, so you fear that every cough, sneeze, hiccup, etc. is going to be the one that does you in. Forget cancer – you're going to die by way of toddler snot.

There you go! Everything you need to know about the next few months of your life! And they all lived happily ever after. What's that? You feel jipped? Fiiine…Here's some more detail for you; let's go back to the beginning.

* * *

The first chemo session will feel very strange. You'll walk into the blood draw, same as you have in the past, but today will feel different. In one way, you will feel a bit excited. Then you may feel weird for feeling excited. *Am I masochistic?* you'll think to yourself. Who in their right mind would be excited for this? I think you should be excited! This is the first step in the next part of your journey, and you can't finish what you don't start, right? But it's not a normal excited. It's the excited where your hands shake a little bit. You'll sit in the chair, anxiously awaiting the next step. When the nurse puts the rubber tourniquet on your arm, your hand will instantly go cold, and you'll be smacked with the reality of a 21-gauge needle. Breathe. I found it best **not to** watch the preparation, and **to watch** as the needle was inserted into my arm. This took away any element of surprise and mitigated a flinch that would make the nurse start over.

Oh, pre-cancer, I hated needles so bad! At one of my first blood draws, I was so anxious that my fist clenched and flexed the muscles in my arm to a point where the nurse couldn't get the needle into my vein. By the time I was able to relax, we could have been done! The nurse will make small talk, and through the cottonmouth, you'll let her know that it's your first chemo session. She'll smile at you with knowing eyes and reassure you that everything will go smoothly. And it will.

Eventually you'll make it into the chemo room, and they'll sit you in a comfortable chair. I imagine there are a ton of different setups depending where you are, but Miami Cancer Institute erred on the side of privacy and had recliners set apart with curtains, kind of like a television emergency room. The floor was quiet, except for the incessant beeping and there was little conversation. My 8'x8' medical oasis even had a chair for my guest. From what I'm told, it wasn't very comfortable. I would come to turn my recliner to face out the window, toward a really nice fountain as part of the routine. A decent sightline for live-action poisoning.

Once the drugs arrive from the pharmacy – cook to order, they are - the nurse will insert the needle into the port and flush it out with saline. This is one of the most surreal feelings I have ever experienced. The first time they do it is something that will be forever burned into your memory.

A quick aside about the port... The port is a small (I assume it's small) catheter that is inserted during your mastectomy surgery, under your skin, that has a tube straight into your heart. The chemo drugs are pumped through this so that their acidic nature doesn't rubberize your veins. Also, since it's relatively permanent, it's durable. In a strange way, it's comfortable. I highly recommend that if given the option, you decide to utilize the port.

So, there you are – the nurse is about to flush your port. Take it from me, put some gum in your chemo bag and pop a brand-new piece as the nurse is preparing the port area. You'll instantly feel cold, then you'll go flush. Then you'll get this extremely weird, salty-metallic taste in your mouth. It's disgusting and will make you nauseous. Chew that gum, sister!

Once they flush your port, they'll give you pre-chemo drugs. These drugs may vary, but their main goal is to ensure that your body is prepared to take the chemo. I had a lovely cocktail of anti-nausea, anti-inflammatory and steroids, which made me uber talkative. Like clockwork, within 10 minutes of receiving the steroids, I was rambling to whichever parent was in the room about God only knows what.

Immediately following the pre-chemo drugs, they moved on to the chemo drugs. Within minutes I would be out like a light, a nice reprieve for my parents from the rambling, and four hours later it would be over. It was very strange that I would wake up on my own about 10 minutes before the whole thing was done. I wonder if there was a sedative of some sort mixed in, or if this was just my body preserving my mind. But all in all, it was a relatively simple procedure.

As I write this, I am imagining what comes next: removing the needle – and it can still feel it. I shudder because it's another one of those awkward feelings, where it incites nausea and chest tightening, but for no real reason. Maybe it was the sound, maybe the location since I couldn't see what they were doing (my port was just below my collarbone on the right side of my chest) – either way, it's another one of those burned-into-the-memory events.

So, chemo itself isn't so bad. Sure, it's time consuming, and there are some small bouts of nausea and weird, immediate side effects, but overall, the process is fairly seamless.

I know what you're thinking… "Fuck you, Jessica. How can you say chemo isn't that bad? I can't believe you have the nerve to put it out into the world that chemo has been overhyped and under-understood for…ever. You have some audacity to share a story that isn't really even a 'story' at all…is it?"

I know! I said that to myself the entire time. It's not lost on me that I had it relatively easy – in hindsight at least. I mean, while this was taking place, I just took it one day at a time, not knowing what the next day would bring. I battled with the concept of how this could possibly be so different from what I've seen others go through – what I've seen on television… But, I had to ask myself: what exactly did you expect, Jess? What did you want to happen? Did you want to be sick as a dog, vomiting all day and night 'as seen on tv'? Did you want to look drawn and pale and 'sick'? No, of course not.

Have you ever noticed that they (the proverbial 'they,' read: TV writers) never tell you the name of the chemo drugs? And they don't show you the entire session. They don't even show you the port or the needle…I mean, c'mon. It's TELEVISION! For one, as I mentioned before, chemo is boring.

Secondly, television writers are paid to incite predictable emotions from the audience that their advertisers are hoping to will cause women, ages 25-54 to buy tampons, White Claws, Poise pads and the newest wrinkle cream. Their jobs depend on viewers getting emotional and weepy, otherwise, they won't be vulnerable enough to give in to the marketing messages that come during the 16 minutes of commercials in your one-hour airing of insert-prime-time-television-drama-here.

But, separately, and in all seriousness, when you visit the treatment center prior to your first session, the nurses and doctors will try to prepare you based on the notion that, in theory, the next few months of your life could feel like the world is about to end. They'll tell you about every possible side effect that any statistically significant number of test subjects has ever experienced. They'll tell you that you'll likely get sick, you'll be fairly lethargic and depending on the type of chemo drugs you've been prescribed, a litany of other drug-specific possibilities. I blame this need for CYA *(cover your ass)* on the overly litigious society in which we live.

I had my eight rounds of chemo split between two separate regimens. For the first four treatments, I had an infusion of Adriamycin and Cytoxan, and the second set of four was Taxol. The pre-chemo session had me believing that I'd be pukey and all but dead for the first four sessions, and that the second half of chemo should be a cake walk in comparison. They told me nausea should set in pretty quickly and stick around for a while. I would most likely experience a metallic taste in my mouth for the duration, and I'd lose my taste completely for some of my favorite foods and drinks. I'd definitely lose my hair, but not for approximately three treatments. They also warned me about a hundred other possibilities.

With the Adriamycin and Cytoxan cocktail (also known as *The Red Devil)*, I was sick on day one...sort of. On the day of chemo #1, as well as the day after, anytime I was just sitting around, I would instantly feel nauseous. I was three weeks removed from major surgery, and two weeks removed from fertility preservation, so suffice it to say that all I was doing was sitting around. So I thought I would try going for a walk around my neighborhood. That seemed to alleviate the nausea, but it didn't make logical sense to me. Was I really even nauseous? Once I asked myself that question, I challenged myself that the next time it happened (the nausea), I would hold out and let myself vomit. But it never happened. In fact, I came to realize that all the preparation they had given me had really just led to phantom symptoms. I didn't vomit one time during four months of chemo. I only became nauseous first thing in the morning, on an empty stomach, but as soon as I ate something, I was fine. Like...FINE.

I was extremely tired but was able to make it through most days without a nap. I'd go to bed early and sleep late, but my body was still healing. I never experienced the metallic taste, but I did lose my taste for some of my favorites. No more Coca-Cola. No more McDonalds or Chipotle. No more milk, but ice cream and cheese were alive and well in my diet. I experienced dry, hot cottonmouth. I craved mostly cold foods and drinks, so I found myself on a smoothie and Frappuccino diet. Still, I tried to eat healthy and drink as much water as I could manage.

My hair began to fall out quickly – and I decided early on that I would be prepared. I purchased a wig – or as they call it for insurance purposes, a *cranial prosthetic* – and was hell-bent on keeping as much control over my body as possible. I wasn't going to be a victim to the chemo eating through my hair follicles. I'd go bald on my terms. More to come on that later.

I suffered from extreme itching during the Adriamycin and Cytoxan regimen. I experienced this mostly in my hands and feet. I also experienced these symptoms in areas where my skin creased and sweat accumulated, for example, behind my knees, my arm pits, the forearm side of my elbows and my groin. This itching was extremely embarrassing. It's not so bad to have itchy hands and be able to subtly scratch the itch away, but everywhere else starts to look extremely awkward. Out of all the things I was dealing with and going through, there was no reason to have been embarrassed, but nonetheless, I was. When I raised this to my doctors, they told me that while annoying, this was completely normal, and yet another side effect of chemo. Drinking water helped, but it wasn't a game changer. Even prescription topical ointment wasn't enough to subside the itching and I found myself tearing through the skin, even with my paper-thin fingernails. I still have scars in the meaty parts between my thumbs and forefingers on both hands.

One side effect that I was actually looking forward to was having my period stop during chemo. Might as well appreciate the silver lining, right? From being like clockwork pre-cancer, my monthly menstrual cycle stopped immediately after my first chemo session and stayed gone for a year almost to the day. It was pretty amazing, but to be honest, with everything else going on, I almost didn't even notice. However. The side effect to that side effect, or maybe the more scientific root cause of that side effect, is that chemo put me into perimenopause, which is the purgatory before full-blown menopause. Will it come back or not? Am I still ovulating? Do I even have any more eggs to pump out? Where are my hormones and what are they up to? Why is it so hot in here? The minute my period stopped, I went headfirst into hot flashes.

I don't care what the movies show you, in my opinion, they're liars. Maybe for some women, menopause is indeed her sitting at the breakfast table, reading the paper in white linen pants and a blue denim-ish blouse, while her aging husband fans her ever so delicately with the day's newspaper. For me, it was sitting at my desk, in an office that was already set to 70 degrees, with a desk fan on full force, and a tissue in-hand to blot my forehead from the rolling beads of sweat that made it look like we were in the rice patties of Vietnam. It was having perfectly styled hair go from airy and flowing to an out-of-the-shower, get-me-a-towel, matted, wet mess in a matter of seconds. It was wearing nothing but black so that me sweating through my sports bra wasn't visible to anyone. It was terrible, uncontrollable, embarrassing and unfair.

I spoke to both of my grandmothers and my mom about their menopause experiences and none of them had it quite like that. Maybe they were stronger than I was, or maybe they had simply come to terms with it because theirs all played out on a more natural schedule. Regardless, nothing helped these feelings, and the hot flashes continued long after chemo was over. Finally, they subsided for the most part once my period came back, but my body temperature hasn't been the same since.

The hot flashes and itching brought on a different level of stress, which was compounded by the hair loss and I felt strange. My eyebrows and eyelashes were almost completely gone, and I decided that it was best to go ahead and pluck the few remaining hairs. I was gutted. I was fine with losing my head hair, and it was great not having to shave my legs! But, losing my eyebrows and eyelashes – especially my eyelashes – was downright debilitating. Ugh it sounds so stupid to write...*debilitating*...Jesus! Forget the two, 8-inch long scars on my chest, or the fact that I had zero breast tissue...*I didn't have eyelashes! WAAA!*

Aside from my boobs, these were the part of my body that I felt made me most feminine. My eye lashes were long and full, and even with no mascara gave me a glammed-up aesthetic. At this point, my head was bald, my face was bald, and the lack of contrast just made me look like a blank canvas. When I first lost my hair, there were some cosmetics brands that were offering tutorials, specifically to cancer patients. I did a short session at Sephora prior to losing my eyebrows so that I would be able to draw them on once they fell out. Honestly, I spent about $50 on makeup that I never used, but the feeling of being prepared was invaluable to me.

The Taxol – phase two of chemo – was supposed to be the easy one. Not for me. This one kicked my ass. The hot flashes continued, but the itching thankfully subsided. Luckily, I still wasn't nauseous.

However, I had bone and joint pain to rival a 90-year-old woman with arthritis. This wasn't the type of joint pain that you have forever from playing soccer into your teens. This was the type that made me walk around my apartment on the balls of my feet, looking like a velociraptor. Arms tucked in tight to my body, knees bent, trying to make myself small and light. It was horrific. I spent these days on the couch, under a blanket, hoping chemo brain didn't make me forget something more than an arm's reach away.

I had pains in bones that I didn't even think of as bones. It sounds dumb, I know, but how does one actually get pain in the sternum or the femur? I have no clue, but trust me, it happens because the largest, densest bones in your body are the ones that produce white blood cells through the bone marrow inside. You know when you have to crack your knuckles? That's what it felt like...but with no actual joint. It's mind-blowing to me to this day how my bones could feel compressed and like they were expanding – like a metal pipe in a vice and an Easter Peep in the microwave...at the same time.

Oddly enough, the treatment for this pain is Claritin – yup, the allergy medicine. Though it worked fairly well, it took a little while to kick in. Once you've felt this pain, it doesn't matter how quickly the medicine works, or how much of the pain it takes away, you're still drained once it's gone; and for me, only sleeping through the night was strong enough to cleanse my memory palate.

As an extreme 'thinker,' the worst side effect for me was chemo brain. Normally sharp as a tack, an elephant in terms of memory, and a human calculator, I found myself without words and stumbling over simple math. There were times when I would be talking normally and then just stop. The words would cease to fire, and I didn't even realize it. It was as if I hadn't even been speaking at all. People would look at me funny and I would shrug it off. One time someone explained it to me, and I was mortified. I hadn't even realized it was happening. I did notice little blips like giving a cashier ten dollars instead of $15 to cover the $12 grocery bill, or even forgetting where I put my sneakers (they were on my feet) or forgetting a conversation from 10 minutes ago. It was extremely difficult for me to accept these types of changes, but there was nothing I could do. Public service warning: three years out of chemo, and I still occasionally suffer from chemo brain.

One set of side effects that I don't remember being told about was the sensitivity in my eyes and nose. From the second or third treatment, I experienced an extremely keen sense of smell. When I would go for walks, I swear that if eight dogs had used the same tree to relieve themselves, I could smell all eight urine varieties individually. Let's just say, this did not help keep the nausea away. It was disgusting and my sniffer hasn't really gone back to 'normal.'

My eyes were another story. I had expected to have vision problems, and for the first time ever in life, I had to get glasses. But separate from the onset of blurred vision, my eyes were all of a sudden really sensitive to light, and worse, water. Sunglasses were required anytime I was outside, even if it was early morning or dusk. Any fractal of natural light that hit my eyes sans shades would all but blind me and cause them to water incessantly.

I should have known this would be a dumb idea (and yes, I was warned), but one weekend during my four-month fling with chemo, I was over in Tampa with my Bowl Week crew and we all took a dip in a hotel swimming pool. As careful as I was not to go underwater, I somehow got some chlorinated water in my eyes. Like, seriously, a single drop must have rolled down off my head from an errant splash, and with no eyebrows to stop it, it was game over for me. The reaction I had to that one drop of pool water was so bad that one of my friends had to walk me to my hotel room and guide me to the shower. There I stood for 10 very cold minutes trying to peel my eyelids from my eyeballs. Or so it felt. I couldn't open my eyes for longer than a couple of seconds without them feeling like they were rolling back into my head, so I went to sleep. The next day, I looked high as a kite, but thankfully, I felt fine. TIP: Don't even risk going swimming while on chemo.

I'm not sure if it's right to even try to separate Chemo from its side effects, but I think it's an important designation as I sit here, thinking back. The body is such an amazing organism. These side effects happened, and when they did, they were in full force; but I could feel my body fighting for normalcy. I could feel the never give up attitude in my gut and so it happened that every week during my four months of chemo was different. I was always trying to use my waking hours to stay as busy and distracted as possible. That seemed to work for me, but when push comes to shove, you will absolutely need to find your own happy medium.

CHAPTER
TWELVE

IDENTITY

On the morning of Tuesday, April 4, 2017, I woke up at the crack of dawn to make sure my dad and I would have time to grab Starbucks before heading over to Miami Cancer Institute for Chemo #2. I see that look on your face – this is a no judgment zone! We had done this week one of chemo and that treatment went smoothly, so I wasn't going to test superstition. In case you're wondering, I also had a chemo uniform. Every week, it was exactly the same thing: hot pink socks that had R & L markings on the appropriate feet (just in case chemo brain got the best of me), gray or black track pants, a black sports bra and a black tank top that read "Challenge Accepted" across the bust. It was my power suit, my cape and my badge of honor all rolled into one.

My parents had decided to switch off on who went to chemo with me. The deal was that the lucky one of any given week would head down to Miami the night before and spend the night. I'd buy Starbucks before chemo in the morning and they'd buy lunch afterwards. On this morning, like many mornings, we talked about how everything was going as we ordered my Frappuccino and my dad's boring coffee.

We were a bit early on that day, so we sat and enjoyed our coffees at Starbucks for a bit, rather than adding any extra time to our day at MCI. I told him how things seemed to be going well, and that I was worried about when my hair would start to fall out. It wasn't supposed to start falling out until after the third treatment, but I had begun to notice more than the normal shedding on my pillow at night, as well as in the shower. He empathized with me, but reminded me that it wouldn't be permanent, and then cracked a joke or two about how he shouldn't jinx it because he was still waiting for his to grow back. My dad is very bald. It was a joke I had heard a thousand times, but today, at 7am sitting in Starbucks, it was downright funny. I told him that when the time came, I'd probably shave my head on a live stream, and he looked at me like I was nuts.

The next few hours were nothing new. We waited, I got hooked up. I rambled then fell asleep. He played on his iPad. At one point, my constantly running mind got the better of me and when I woke up, the tone of the day changed.

"Do you have time to swing by the salon after this? What if I do it today?" I asked.

He gave me that look again. "What? Wait. Seriously?"

I tugged on a few strands of hair at the top of my forehead, expecting resistance, and they came right out, like a handful of weeds from very loose soil. I think he was as surprised as I was that it came out so easily, as his jaw dropped open a bit. I could tell it was sinking in – that this was real.

"Welp, today it is," I told him, "I'll lose my hair on my terms. Cancer isn't taking this from me too." And we headed to the on-site boutique as soon as I was unplugged.

My dad was on camera duty for the Facebook Live. After he got accustomed to my Android, it took about 32 minutes from the time we started recording to the end of the video, but it felt like an eternity. I narrated the entire process, with short interludes from the stylist about the process and importance of this step and the subsequent trims.

As your hair grows back – eventually – it's going to house remnants of all the chemo drugs and other chemicals, so it's imperative that you keep it trimmed to maintain its overall health. Eventually, all the drug-hair will grow out. I already had short hair, so the idea of no hair wasn't as drastic for me as it might have been for someone accustomed to long, luscious locks. Talk to your doctor about whether or not you can expect to lose your hair during chemo (everyone's treatments are different). If there is a decent probability, I highly recommend taking the initiative to ease into the new you. Go ahead and cut your hair a few times before it falls out, dramatically shorter each time.

I sat in the chair at the salon, and was surprised that the process was less dramatic than I originally expected. Britney circa 2007 was what I had in mind – you know, clippers straight to the scalp. But no, my stylist cut most of my hair off with scissors before ultimately cleaning it up with the buzzer. Anticlimactic to say the least.

As many of you know, Facebook Live allows for real-time commenting by viewers. My dad kept me up to speed with the audience's reactions and comments, but I challenged myself not to face the mirror until the very end. That was a difficult 20 minutes!

At about five minutes in, I realized that I hadn't brought any makeup with me, nor had I worn any that day. (Let's be honest, I never wore makeup to chemo.) Hair and cheekbones – those are what make you look feminine without makeup, and it's interesting how much your haircut actually draws attention to your cheekbones. Learn from my mistake: bring your makeup with you the day you decide to 'smooth cut' your head!

For the most part, actually cutting my hair wasn't an unbearably emotional experience, but there were a few moments that brought the waterworks. Once I realized – as did others, evidenced by their comments on the live feed – that I closely resembled my late brother, it was very tough to keep it together. I still hadn't seen myself in the mirror, but I could only imagine. I've come to find out that we share the same head shape, hairline and cowlick.

Overall, shaving my head when I did, and on my terms, was a very liberating experience and I'm glad that I kept that piece of control! Control or not though, having my dad there with me that day was so important. It's okay to be vulnerable and to need or want someone to go through these milestones with you. Just remember you don't have to do any of it alone!

As I was having my hair cut that day, my stylist told me a story about a conversation she had with one of the doctors, where he just couldn't understand how a cancer patient's first words after getting the news that she'd have to undergo chemotherapy and radiation was, "Am I going to lose my hair?" She told me, "They (read: men) just can't comprehend it – these women weren't asking about surgery or implants or remedies for vomiting; they were asking if they'd lose their hair."

As women, we put so much emphasis on our hair and our looks in general – to a point where it becomes part of our identity. Growing up, I kept my hair long so that I could have a ponytail like all the other soccer girls. But by high school, I had cut it short. I saw it as a functional approach to the south Florida heat and my indifference toward fashion in favor of ease-of-use. As I got older and more self-aware, I started to care a bit more. Eventually for me, short hair said I'm confident enough to say "Fuck You" to social norms and expectations. It also said, "Man, it's hot out there. This is so functional!" This time, however, was obviously a different situation.

The first couple days of baldness were a bit of an adjustment, as you feel every little thing. Every draft, every drop of water…such a crazy sensation! As I continued on through the chemo process, my head got extremely sensitive, probably from the hair follicles being zapped by the drugs. Sleeping was once again unbearable – even the gentlest touch of my head to the pillow was torture. I ended up purchasing head scarves that were like long, super soft shirt sleeves, and these seemed to stay put and do the job while I slept. For days that I had to be or chose to be out in the sun, I bought wide headbands and wore a ball cap.

I was very lucky that I was confident enough in newly exposed shape of my head to go through my days, sans wig. Once I saw that I could pull off the buzz cut, I decided to rock it, telling myself that only once my hair fell out completely, would I put my $300 investment to use.

Before I knew it, every shower yielded more and more stubble in my hands; and every morning I woke up to more and more scruff on my pillow. The first morning was fairly disturbing, but like everything else, I was soon desensitized to the molting that was out of my control.

I pride myself on being relatively self-aware, but self-awareness is by definition in the eye of the beholder. Case in point, one day after all of my hair had fallen out and I was bald, bald, I was getting out of my car in a shopping center (probably on my way into HomeGoods or TJMaxx) and I was startled when I saw someone in the car parked next to mine. He looked back at me with my same horrified look. I quickly realized it was my own reflection in the car window. I laughed out loud! Then emotion overcame me, and I didn't know what else to do except get back in my car and cry. So, I did – I beat the steering wheel, mumbled through spit to myself and cried big, heavy tears. And then I was done; melt down over. Nothing a little retail therapy couldn't fix…how convenient!

The wig I purchased felt like a helmet and added at least another 10 degrees to the summer heat; and even in all its blonde-highlighted, face-framing glory, it wasn't me. I opted not to wear it on most occasions, and on the few that I did (maybe once or twice over the course of 2017), I was more self-conscious than without it. In fact, this $300 cranial prosthetic has seen more daylight in the years following my cancer journey than it did during. Happy Halloween, everybody!

Originally, I had planned to do a super creative "Wig Reveal" event since everyone and their mother seemed to be hosting gender reveal parties at the time. I was going to set up a fake press conference with four ridiculous wigs on mannequin heads spaced equally across the table, similar to College Football's signing day. Like all my other videos, this would be hosted on Facebook Live and I would speak in depth about each wig and what it brought to the table (literally in this case), what was going through my head as each one made its way into my very own final four. The high point of the presser would be the final reveal, where I would don the wig for the first time in public. But by the time I had selected my wig, cut off my hair, had the wig trimmed, and ultimately decided I wasn't even going to wear it, the Wig Reveal had lost its allure. I just didn't care, and that video never made its debut.

CHAPTER
THIRTEEN

RECONSTRUCTION

My last chemo treatment was on July 6, 2017, a mere five months and five days after my initial diagnosis, and I was elated when my post-treatment blood work came back favorable. My body was officially on the mend, and since my white blood cells were replenishing themselves and cancelling the designation of being *immunocompromised*, my Plastic Surgeon was finally able to resume the tissue expanding process.

The doctor was able to inflate the tissue expanders with just over 100ccs of saline before chemo started and the risk of infection became too high. Afterward, I began to see him weekly to add another 100ccs each time, and by the third time, he deemed me ready to schedule the reconstruction: Friday,

August 11th would be the day that the 500-pound gorilla would finally get off my chest and be replaced by three and a half pounds of silicone.

By the time I went in for surgery, the expanders had been filled to just over 500ccs of saline, which created enough give in the muscle and skin to accommodate an 800cc, round, high-profile silicone implant. The doctor would use the original incision scars to remove the expanders and replace them with the implants. He would reduce the scars as much as possible upon closing and would also remove my chemo port.

I haven't spoken too much about my Plastic Surgeon, but he was phenomenal. I don't think I could have asked for anyone better. Aside from being an attractive Latino (a bit of eye candy is always nice), he took the time to listen to me, my concerns and my goals, but also laid out my options in a way such that I ultimately chose correctly. Surely, had I decided to go with a different shape, number of ccs or profile, he would have obliged, but by the time I left with my surgical plan, I wasn't sure how many – if any – of the decisions were actually mine. It didn't matter. I was uber confident in his judgement and abilities, and I was glad to have the guidance.

Once again, #MySaintlyParents came down for the surgery, but aside from them being there at the hospital, I remember nothing at all after I started counting backward from 10 on the operating table.

10…9…Saturday.

With the memories from the mastectomy still pretty fresh in my head, I went into recovery pretty optimistic. It's funny how your perspective changes. By August, being poked and prodded and touched was so commonplace, none of it phased me at all. Except for the drains. Fucking drains. Like the Backstreet Boys, there were back again, but at least this time I had some experience. The...we'll call it 'output' wasn't quite as gross or plentiful as the first time around and they were out within a week. Yay, healing!

I had always been relatively content with my boobs pre-cancer, but given the opportunity, I opted for the largest implant available. As I discussed this with my doctor, I was comforted by his openness and candor. Pre-surgery I was a solid C-cup, and normally, putting 800ccs under that would put me among the ranks of a Dolly or a Pam. However, without any breast tissue at all post-mastectomy, this size would make me look very proportionate and the volume would fill out my frame very well.

Today, I'm a true to size D-cup, and I have zero regrets regarding the size selection. I deal with a bit of neck and back pain from the weight, but I'm very scared to do any sort of strength training on my pectoral muscles. I've attempted pushups, but the slightest twinge in my chest makes me feel like I need to vomit. Between the lack of feeling in the breast itself, the contraction of the muscle on top of an obviously foreign object and the fear of the unknown, I'd rather leave my boobs alone. I'm sure there are perfectly safe exercises you can find online, but I'm just not interested in any sort of risk that will screw them up, so I'll deal with a little bit of discomfort.

My reconstruction really looks phenomenal (this time I am bragging), but sometimes I get so mad at myself. Every now and then, I'll be getting in the shower and stop to stare at my naked breasts. They look funny – different from how I remember. They're wide-set and I can see the scars. Before 3 minutes pass, I'm already planning a nip here and a tuck there, as if it's just part of the routine. *How greedy*, I think to myself. *THIS. WAS. NOT. A. BOOB. JOB. You are one of the lucky ones that was graced with two phenomenal surgeons.* As I wrote this book, I was doing research – finally Googling – and came across before and after photos of random, anonymized women. My God, I was so fortunate, and I thank my lucky stars that I came through this looking as anatomically 'normal' as I did.

My thanksgiving for the normality that I received does not downplay the feelings you may be having regarding your own surgery, and it shouldn't put any additional fear in your head. As you move into this part of the process and begin to make these decisions (if you decide to do reconstruction at all), you need to assess and be at peace with your goals.

I was 32 and single when I made these decisions. From my point of view, future conversations would be hard enough having to explain my history with cancer in the first place, so I wanted to at least try to avoid the shock factor the first time Mr. Right took off my bra. I remember discussing this insecurity with an old friend. As I described the way my chest looked and expressed my fears about how any guy who sees this would cut and run, his face grimaced. He said to me, "Look, if some douchebag is going to do that, fuck 'em. You beat fucking cancer. Those scars are a badge of honor." Whoa. Also, marry me!

Listen to your Plastic Surgeon and really have an honest conversation with him or her about what you can expect and what you want to avoid. If you have a particular aesthetic in mind, tell them – give them a goal. They won't risk overpromising and underdelivering. They will tell you if what you're asking for in unrealistic or unachievable. Make your decisions and move on. Don't second guess anything, but if I may give you my two cents (hey, you've already come this far!), go just a little bit bigger than what you initially think you want.

CHAPTER
FOURTEEN

FINISHING TOUCHES

For a long time after the reconstruction, I contemplated some of the options I had regarding nipples. For now, they were replaced by 8-inch long, dark pink scars, stretching straight across the center of both breasts. I was torn. While being extremely self-conscious about their appearance, I was hell bent on leaving well enough alone. I looked at pictures online to see what other women had done. If you are curious, and only after your reconstruction is complete, go to Google or Pinterest and search 3D nipple tattoos, or Mastectomy tattoo. Remember: there's a reason my surgeon told me not to Google anything and there are images of horror stories out there that you don't need to see.

I was impressed by the beauty and creativity of some of these tattoos. Some women opted to tattoo a full corset, while others used flowers and beautiful, powerful, meaningful imagery to mask their scars. Some opted for very anatomically correct 3D nipples, while others reimagined them as hearts or flowers. They were stunning and bold and fierce, but my jury was still out. I was in no rush and did not want to make a decision I'd regret. I'm no stranger to tattoos and I knew myself: if and/or when the time was right, I'd go ahead and pull the trigger.

By this time, my hair was starting to grow back. One thing about new hair that I was told but didn't quite comprehend was that in a lot of cases, the hair grows back very different from the original color, texture and manageability. For example, before chemo, my hair was dark brown with a little bit of gray starting to peek through at my temples and was relatively straight. It would hold a curl or a wave if I tried really hard and used enough product. However, it grew back extremely curly – think Labradoodle – and dark gray with a white – what I like to call – *halo* around my face.

I decided to let it grow out and see if the weight of the hair would straighten itself out. It didn't. My head got bushier and bushier, growing bulbous rather than sleek. After having lost it all, as ridiculous as it sounds, I didn't want to cut it at all and so for almost a year, I let it grow wild. Who was I to tempt fate? However, after seeing photos from my sister's wedding, I finally decided to dye it and have it cut and styled.

I dyed it at home one Saturday morning and broke down in tears when I stepped out of the shower and I saw *myself* in the mirror. I looked like me. Leading up to that moment, I didn't realize just how much my new hair had contributed to my overall look. I didn't realize the toll that the dull, dark gray color had taken on me, making me feel so alien to myself.

Once it was dyed, I scheduled the first possible appointment with my stylist. She took me in that weekend and proved her rock star status. I don't know how she did it, or if maybe it was just *time*, but my hair's texture was all of a sudden closer to normal than it had been in almost two years. Thankfully, it has maintained the new texture, and I've even noticed that it's healthier than ever before. If there's a silver lining, it's that losing my hair to chemo gave me a hard reset on all the damage I had done to it over the years.

In that process of finally coming to terms with the new texture of my hair, and subsequently getting it almost 100% back to normal, I was starting to gain more and more confidence and moxie than I ever realized I had lost. So, after over a year of being haunted by the scars every day while letting my new body settle into itself, I decided I was finally ready to do something with my bare breasts. At the recommendation of my Plastic Surgeon, I chose a tattoo artist who specialized in 3D nipple tattoos[7] for survivors; and on May 25, 2018, I had her put the *anatomically correct* finishing touches on my new normal.

As you go through these stages, take some time to yourself and remember to breathe. As my trusted circle of pre-release readers read this book, many of them commented that they never knew I was feeling certain ways, or that I went through some of these emotions or steps to finally being okay at all. It's okay not to be okay all the time. You are going to have your own emotions and your own reactions to your own experiences. Take them in stride, make decisions only when you actually have decisions to make, and remember that you're a strong, sane, powerful human that can handle anything you decide to handle, however and whenever you decide to handle it. Just keep going.

---

[7] Be sure to do some research with your insurance company regarding the financial allotment for the tattoos. There may be additional paperwork for you and the artist to complete in order to be reimbursed for the work.

PART II

EMOTIONAL

CHAPTER
FIFTEEN

PART II: BEFORE YOU CONTINUE

I split this book into two parts because you're going to naturally compartmentalize the situation with which you're faced. Your medical decisions will become robotic and you will go through the motions to get done what you need to get done as quickly as possible in order to beat this thing. You'll likely deal with the emotions separately.

This next section will seem markedly different from Part I. In Part II, I'm going to share with you some of the emotions and experiences that stick out in my memory. As I wrote this, I was actually pretty surprised at the bits that were etched in my brain. In some cases, they haunt me a bit, and in others, they inspire me and push me forward, whether the situation is related to cancer or not.

As you'll read in the following chapters, there are so many things I thought I had already figured out, or that I had already dealt with, but that came rushing back at random trigger-points during my cancer journey. Sometimes they were debilitating; sometimes they were irrational; sometimes they manifested in humor or anger or fear or empowerment.

I'm excited to share my stories, learnings, tips, and life lessons with you. My goal here is that you come away from this book knowing that the emotions you're going to experience – whatever they are and whenever they come to you – during your journey are normal, will vary day to day and are something to embrace and learn from.

My stories are meant to empower and inspire you, so while I will definitely keep them real, I always look for the lesson or the silver lining or the positive mindset. But cancer is a big deal. A big, shitty, annoying, infuriating, painful clusterfuck of emotions. And you don't have to deal with it on your own. Please, if you feel overwhelmed or depressed or anxious, talk to someone – a friend, family member, a support group, or maybe even a therapist or social worker.

CHAPTER
SIXTEEN

WARRIOR

A few weeks ago, I ordered pizza to my house. I had some friends over and between the conversation, passing hours and alcohol, we needed some food (read: carbs). As the delivery driver pulled up to the security gate at the front of the development, she called me from her personal cell phone and asked how to get in. I had forgotten to put the code for the callbox on the delivery instructions. I proceeded to give her the number: "It's star, number, number, number, pound." She didn't understand, and in broken English, asked me to repeat the code. Given my cusp-of-millennial demographic group, I used my I-took-four-years-in-high-school-and-two-in-college-level Spanish and repeated, "Es estrella, numero, numero, numero, uhhhh pound sign." I could hear her dial 4 keys…then a pause. Shit – got it! "Estrella, numero, numero, numero, *hashtag*." Open Sesame!

Ahhh, hashtags. Throughout the social media evolution, or revolution as it were, what used to be a literal metadata tagging notation within the codebase of a website, or simply a pound sign to us layfolk, became commonplace on platforms like Twitter, Instagram and eventually Facebook. Apparently at some point during the dawn of social media, someone somewhere decided that everything needed a label. Cue choirs of angels! Thus was born the hashtag that we know and (I) use incorrectly today.

In some – maybe most – cases, hashtags have legitimate value. You want to see all the photos people took at your wedding and posted to their personal social media accounts? Search for the strategically created hashtag. You want to see what topics are trending around the world in order to stay current on the latest and greatest feud or social cause? Search for or browse the hashtags. You want to be a part of that movement? Use the designated hashtag.

Hashtags have become a social status symbol: random, globalized groups of people yearning for some sort of acceptance or inclusion. To be a part of something. Or to be heard, seen or read: "Look at me! I'm hip – I used a hashtag. I'm part of something. I have a purpose." These hashtags while sometimes very witty, funny or downright literal have become the Kleenex or Band-Aid of the social media era – so commonplace, misused or overused that they hold almost no meaning and ultimately dilute the brand or the root message they at one time aimed to serve. An inside joke. A secret handshake.

For those who know and understand, sure, there's a lot of meaning. For those who are not part of the in crowd, there's a whole cycle that ensues: misuse, shame, resentment on both sides, apologies, retractions, deletions, repeat.

One of my least favorite hashtags is, or I guess now *used to be*, #WARRIOR. 'Warrior' is the term commonly used for someone who is battling cancer – and it's most commonly used in reference to breast cancer. I guess at some point, someone decided that women needed motivation via a title in order to beat this parasite that is cancer. As if, the diagnosis alone wasn't enough motivation to fight. As if, without associating her identity with a chainmail-clad, weapon-wielding character, she'd have no shot at winning this battle.

Do we really *need* this hashtag? Probably not. Women's bodies are capable of so many amazing feats. We grow humans. We push those humans, who are usually larger than any single part of our own anatomy, out of our bodies through a canal whose normal, resting circumference is that of a boba tea straw. Our biology changes to accommodate providing life-sustaining nutrition to those humans and continues to be able to do so for approximately half our lives. We have the emotional intelligence for empathy and love and care and fear and confidence and bravery and regret all at the same time. We can organize, strategize, optimize, cook, clean, heal and comfort! We don't need your stinkin' chainmail – or your hashtag!

From the day I was diagnosed, I was labeled a #Warrior. At the beginning, I bought in. Probably because I had been conditioned to do so, but as I progressed into the thick of this battle, the term – or at least the way people used it – infuriated me. I had no weapons. I had no army. This was my glorious body fighting against itself. It's such a mind fuck when your body turns on itself. What do you even do with that? I turned to what I knew best.

As I've developed my career over the years, I've read a number of really enlightening, incredibly inspiring business and life-lesson-type books. One of my favorites is *The Seed* by Jon Gordon. Though I feel you should read it for yourself and draw your own conclusions, the premise of this book is that situations will happen in life and work, and regardless of whether you're completely ready to deal with them or not deal with them, to move on or not to move on; regardless of whether it's your decision or not, you have to squeeze every bit of knowledge, insight and experience out of the situation in that moment. More importantly, you do so with the intention of applying it to your next (ad)venture. In the case of cancer, it's possible that you're going to resent your body a bit – especially as you go through chemotherapy and start to have all the side effects. While we've already partially discussed some ways to handle this, I believe that your best bet will be to simply put it out of your mind and compartmentalize as much as possible. There is never going to be a good enough reason for why this happened, and you are never going to be satisfied with any of the lessons you learn along the way. In my experience, it's best to chalk it up to bad luck, and try to find some sort of good in the situation. So that's what I tried to do in this situation. I embraced #Warrior as a battle cry and allowed myself to pivot my feelings along the way – and there were a lot of pivots.

In the beginning, my perception of hashtags and labels and titles regarding the expectations that go along with them was that I was expected to perform. The group that I had created on Facebook[8] for informational purposes had become an audience that I was performing for – a boob-less gladiator in the social media Coliseum. As a #Warrior, it was my job to entertain; to fight; to win. I had to be strong, fearless and steadfast. What people thought was motivational and uplifting was translating as daunting and tiring. (And yes, I'm fully aware that I brought it upon myself.)

One morning while I was preparing for yet another doctor's appointment, I was distracted by Pinterest, and I came across a quote from Sun Tzu's The Art of War (when in Rome, right?):

Victorious warriors win first and then go to war.

Defeated warriors go to war first and then seek to win.

This resonated with me as #Warrior had been such a pain point – a trigger for impostor syndrome. I wasn't special, nor was I trying to be. Again, I was

---

[8] Jess's Cancer-fighting Squad:
https://www.facebook.com/groups/JessCancerFightingSquad/

just trying to survive – to beat this stupid cancer and move on with my life. I wasn't a warrior...I mean, what the hell else was I going to do, lay down and die? C'mon...

If ever there was a cartoon lightbulb to turn on above my head, it was then. I scoffed at myself for giving in to self-pity and made the conscious and deliberate decision to change my perspective. I finally started to see my mental state as the weapon to match my armor for this battle. I certainly did not want to be defeated in my fight against cancer, and according to Sun Tzu, I had to win first – before the battle even started. I realized I had to be victorious in the only place I could be in that time and place: my head. Maybe I was a warrior. Or maybe I just needed to decide to buy into the hype and convince myself that I was.

CHAPTER
SEVENTEEN

ATTITUDE

I would be lying if I told you that I was an angel growing up. I didn't get into actual trouble, or do bad things, but let's just say my grandmothers would describe me as "[having] a mouth on her, that one." I was quick-witted, smart-mouthed and loose-lipped. I was hot-tempered, but cool-mannered, and always respectful of my elders, but quick with a rebuttal and constantly challenging authority. I was sarcastic, relatively funny and with a bit of alcohol (once I was legal, of course), the life of the party.

A self-proclaimed realist, I was a person who was trained early on – either through team sports, or marching band – to think five steps ahead. I was an optimistic leader, but I was pragmatic, strategic and determined. Always in control of, and controll*ing* my future, my psyche, my place and my path in this life.

I learned to tame and temper all of this over the years, mostly with soap in my mouth, a quick backhanded swat, *growing up* in general and reading professional leadership books; but suffice it to say my attitude was never classified as an asset.

And then I got cancer.

In the hour it took to sign in, get called into the exam room, wait for 'the bearer of bad news,' get the bad news, return to my car and melt down, a switch that I didn't even know I possessed had flipped. I'd realize later that this was my infamous attitude finally finding its productive use in my world.

Once I came to terms with the fact that cancer was in my body, it was going to be removed from my body and I would undergo chemotherapy to make sure it never came back into my body, I had to figure out what was next. For maybe the first time in my life, I hadn't seen this step among the five in front of me. And the five I did see were going to have to fit into this new path, not the other way around.

In 2012, shortly after my brother was killed in a motorcycle accident, I uprooted my life and moved to New York.

Wait, wait, wait… Jess, you're telling me your brother was suddenly killed in an accident and your diagnosis was 'maybe the first time' you didn't see that step coming? Surely you could not have foreseen and/or planned for your brother's

accident.

It is 100% true that I hadn't planned on my brother dying suddenly at the age of 24, just a mile or two away from my parents' home in south Florida. But Jimmy's death didn't inherently change my general life plan. He and I were close, sure. He was – is, and will always be – my brother, but at the time of the accident, our lives didn't intersect that much. Mourning, grieving, doing what I could to help my parents and sister through this time was all part of it of course, but that accounted for maybe a month or two of my life. His death, while forcing me to reflect on my relationship with him and with the rest of my family, to analyze and regret that maybe I could have done something circumvent his accident, didn't force my hand.

This circumstance, as horrible as it was, and as much as it's burned into my memory and as much as it drove my outlook on the world, also strengthened me. It made me take off my blinders and realize that I'm not in control of the bigger forces in the universe. It was my first taste of my own mortality and made me realize that none of us are invincible. Naturally, given the self-portrait of my mindset that I gave you a few paragraphs ago, I did what I could to grasp onto the things I did have control over, and continued on the same path I had already begun (climbing the corporate ladder within the advertising industry). Jimmy's death gave me a much-needed kick in the ass and caused me to ask myself, *If not now, when?*

Within three weeks, I found a new job, broke the lease on my Tampa apartment and moved to New York like any self-respecting, rising Advertising industry professional would do. After all, *if I could make it there…*

I lived in New York for two years and in 2014, I flew home over Valentine's Day weekend for a party to celebrate my grandparents' joint 80th birthdays. There were 150 people at the house – all family and close friends – and I realized in the bliss of that moment that my time in New York had run its course. I wanted to be close to everyone again. The last time all of these people had been together was at Jimmy's funeral, and it made me think about how often we wait for something terrible to happen to make a change that we know we need to make.

I thought about Jimmy and how much he would have enjoyed the party. I think I cried that night, realizing for the first time that there were more important things than money and title and climbing the corporate ladder. I spoke to him in my dreams and remembered that his death was one of the main drivers that pushed me to make a tremendous career move – one that would benefit me for the rest of my life, though I didn't know then how. I remembered how though he seemed fun and fancy free, was a light-hearted individual who could make the best out of any situation, and though he wasn't specifically a planner, he always seemed to have some sort of a plan. Even if that plan was flying by the seat of this pants and seeing what would happen.

At the end of the weekend, I flew back to New York, tendered my 6-week notice and began planning the move back home. There are so many emotions that bubble up when major life changes are taking place. I was sad to be leaving this Big Apple dream, but I knew it was the right decision. I was a bit embarrassed that I hadn't *made it there*, but that subsided quickly after late-night beers (and the all-too-normal subsequent Fireball shots) with a close friend. (Is it me or were those cab rides back to Harlem and Washington Heights the highest points of clarity?!) At some point during the night, I had told her that I felt embarrassed that NYC chewed me up and spit me out like it did to so many others. She stopped me and said, "You deciding to be closer to family and move back to Florida is not New York spitting you out. That's you making a decision – adulting, if you will. And since when are you a victim of anything?" I'm paraphrasing, but that's how I remember it.

I thought back to Jimmy's outlook on life – he always believed things would work out. And somehow, they always seemed to do just that. Maybe that's more rose-colored vision, but that's how I choose to remember him. I started evaluating myself and soon realized that in the past two years, I had worked, seen a ton of movies in theaters by myself, worked, drank, worked, mourned over the Jets, attended a couple of fund raisers, and worked. In all my time living in New York, I hadn't lived. Swipe right, baby!

So, I resolved to live. I bought a plane ticket from Miami to London and from Munich to Miami. I'd cross the pond the day after I arrived home in Palm Beach and would be back shortly before my best friend's wedding. Three weeks. No plans. Holy shit.

Try as I did not to plan every detail of this trip (successfully, by the way), I couldn't get the *but then what* out of my head. I was resolved to moving to South Florida and planned to live at home for the foreseeable future, but I didn't have a job. Or health insurance, or anything else lined up. At the time, it seemed as though getting interviews would take forever, so I started applying to jobs about 3 weeks before I left for Europe thinking I could field emails and set up interviews from wherever I happened to be for the weeks following my return stateside.

To my surprise, I started getting calls and interviews right away, and those conversations started teetering on the verge of offer letters. Again, I freaked out. Bird in the hand, I thought. So I called my dad. Should I really even go to Europe? It would be an amazing experience, and probably not one I'd be able to have at any other time in my life. But what about the real world? What if I end these conversations now, and don't get a job when I get back? We talked, and he managed to refrain from lecturing. To be honest, I think I called him expecting (read: wanting) him to tell me that I shouldn't go. That I needed to be an adult and take care of business.

But he didn't try to talk me out of it. He didn't even try that reverse psychology thing he does and that I wised up to circa age 17. (Little does he know; I flipped the script on him years ago.) He simply said, "You know what, Jess? You have the money. You have a place to live when you get back. Go. Don't let this be a *gonnado*⁹. I mean, have you ever NOT landed on your feet?"

And that was that. I went to Europe.

Flash forward a few years and there I was with a shiny new cancer diagnosis and all I could think was, "Have you ever NOT landed on your feet?" Thank God I didn't have foot cancer…that would have been awkward.

I tell this very long story for a couple of reasons. First, it speaks to the notion that I thought I had fully dealt with my brother's death from an emotional perspective, but there were so many points during my fight that I felt him there with me, or thought of him and how he would react or handle individual circumstances. He'd pop into my head at random points, and linger for a bit, just enough to put me at ease. Sometimes him being in my head would challenge me to do better – to try harder – to not give up.

---

⁹ A *gonnado* is a phrase our family (via my dad) coined after my brother died. How many times have you said, "I'm *gonna' (going to) do* this" or "I'm *gonna' do* that"? Whatever the 'this' or 'that' was, that is your *gonnado*.

Cancer bubbled up issues and feelings I thought I had moved past, and it caused me to tie multiple sets of feelings together to come to a grander conclusion, or at least working theory of my life. Experiences and memories and memories of those experiences mold us and prepare us for the next steps in the road. In some ways, although he had been gone for five years, Jimmy helped me get through some of the tougher parts of cancer. The mind is absolutely amazing and frightening at the same time – and sometimes as you're fighting through this, it may scare you a little bit. Let yourself feel, emote, relish in the memories and absorb the in-the-moment clarity. If it's not so clear in the moment, put a pin in it; your mind is sure to bring it full circle.

The second reason I tell this story is because on that trip through Europe, I made some extremely close friends, with whom I stayed in contact over the years. One in particular was from Germany, who I met in London on a walking tour. Shortly after I started chemo, his mother was diagnosed with the same type of breast cancer I had. She was in her 50s, but I was able to be a resource to her during her battle. We emailed back and forth and were each other's cheerleaders. Cancer effects so many people, from all over the world and without bias. It was heartwarming and precious that she and I could help each other out with stories, tips, tricks and encouragement, but none of that would have happened if my life hadn't played out in the course I described.

Every semester, I try to visit my alma mater (#GoBulls) and speak to budding advertising executives – usually juniors and seniors. I talk to them about the real world, what to and not to expect when they graduate; and I give them *Life Lessons According to Jess*. Inevitably, one of the more ballsy students will ask me for tips for planning their impending career. I always tell them some variation of the same story, and it goes something like this:

If I were in your seat right now, and said to myself, "By the time I'm X years old, I want to be a *[insert current title here]*, what should I do?" No matter what I came up with, I'd be wrong. There is no way on earth that I could have planned the way my life would turn out. However, as I stand here now at X years of age, and *[insert current title here]*, and look back at the path I took to get here, it's crystal clear and there's no question that I took the right steps. Every single crazy pivot or tangent or *wouldn't-that-be-cool* opportunity has given me lessons and tools and mental, physical, emotional preparation for the next step. I couldn't have planned it, but it makes total and complete sense. So follow your gut, take the opportunities as they present themselves and don't be afraid to forge your own path. Deep down, you know what is going to work for you, but accept guidance along the way because that too will mold your experience.

We usually use the phrase *Everything happens for a reason* to console people when bad things happen – and rest assured I heard this multiple times when I was diagnosed… But I think everything good happens for a reason too – no matter how small! Chick-fil-A accidentally gave you 12 nuggets instead of eight? Maybe you just needed some extra protein that day! You decide to shirk responsibilities for three weeks, backpack Europe and meet a hot guy in a foreign land? Maybe one day you'll be a resource for his mother's cancer battle…See?

This enlightenment allowed me to embrace the situation and officially decide to offer a positive mindset out to the world. There were some days where I wanted to punch myself in the face for being overly optimistic or for putting on what felt like a façade. It wasn't always sunshine and rainbows, but I was able to redirect that disdain and resentment that I talked about in the last chapter into more productive avenues, or toward what I felt was the greater good. The more I fought the negativity, and the more I resolved to find the good in this particular situation – to try to win the war, the better I felt about the entire predicament. How easy it would have been for me to retreat to sadness, depression and contempt. With this new mindset, there was no doubt that I was in control of my fate. The small seed of optimism and experience was slowly germinating and growing into a pretty positive outlook – something I wasn't really used to. My attitude became an invaluable asset to my recovery, and while I maybe didn't believe it before, *mind over matter* was alive and well.

As a little girl, I was told and reassured that I could do anything I put my mind to; that I could essentially be anything I aspired to be. The day I received my diagnosis and prognosis, I put my mind toward beating cancer and I never second-guessed it. Feelings came and went, but the scales were tipping in my favor, thanks to my mindset. There was no question that I would beat cancer. I was a bad-ass woman that would thrive at all costs. Being a #Warrior and aspiring ultimately to be a #Survivor was 'thriving' at its best.

Accepting and embracing this attitude-as-an-asset mindset is something that will forever impact my life. I hope it is ringing loud and clear through this book and is a paradigm that you can manifest for your future as well.

CHAPTER
EIGHTEEN

MORTALITY

Something happens to you when you're told you have cancer, or when anything devastating happens to you or someone you know. There's a switch that shorts out, igniting a spark of doubt. That spark turns into an ember of disbelief. And that ember turns into a flame of fear, anger and rage. That flame soon ignites a blaze and there is no stopping it. Whether that blaze is one of self-loathing or of self-discovery is completely up to you.

You're forced to look your own mortality straight in the eye. Then one of two things happens: you either say hello and defeatedly welcome it into your life as-is, starting a countdown clock to the day you die; or you tell it to fuck off and thrive in your impending new normal. When I was diagnosed with cancer, I wasn't sure when 'the end' would come, but I didn't want to have any regrets when it did. I looked at my mortality as a challenge of self-discovery:

to live the best life I could; because in the end, or so hundreds of memes on Pinterest have told me, it's the experiences you didn't have that you regret.

I wasn't stupid though. During the first half of my chemo treatments, I played by the doctors' rules. I was very careful about germs and cleanliness, took extreme caution in terms of whom I was around, how I spent my time and what I was exposed to; and I ate and drank as healthy as possible. It was the smart thing to do and I'm glad I took that route. As I've mentioned a few times thus far, I was on an upward career trajectory, and started a new job the Monday before my third chemo session (Tuesday). It made sense to play it safe and make sure I didn't take unnecessary risks, so I'd drive to work, stay in my office as much as possible and drive home. No happy hour, an occasional lunch out, none of the typical Miami cheek kisses to say hello. It was relatively safe, but man, was it boring.

By the time I made it to my final installment of Adriamycin and Cytoxan, I was climbing the walls of my condo and was ready to make some changes. My role at the network included sales strategy and client relations, as well as entertaining, so when I originally took the job, I was expected to travel as needed. For those of you playing along at home, it's strongly advised that chemo patients steer clear of crowded areas and don't subject themselves to enclosed spaces in lieu of fresh air. Long story, short: no airplanes.

I had monitored and analyzed my 'numbers' during the first four treatments. As we've established, I'm no doctor, but I'm pretty good with statistics and math, and so I decided the odds were in my favor. I informed my doctors – the Medical Oncologist and the Plastic Surgeon – that I had no intention of being grounded for another four rounds, and, reluctantly, they talked me through what I needed to know. They provided suggestions to stay as safe as possible and gave me a just-in-case prescription for antibiotics. Should my fever spike above 100.7 degrees, I was to go directly to the emergency room regardless of what city I was in, give them my medical history and be quarantined until further notice. I could not miss scheduled bloodwork or chemo treatments, so I would have to be very strategic with my travel planning. As far as the tissue expanders were concerned, the Plastic Surgeon reassured me that any change in altitude would not affect them, so I was all set (#TheMoreYouKnow). As far as I was concerned, all of these warnings and recommendations were small potatoes. Everything was going to be perfectly fine.

I went through the next two months on a plane out of town at least twice a month. Go big or go home, right? (It's important to note that my company in no way, shape or form required me to travel. This was a decision that I made on my own and whose consequences I brought upon myself.) During one span, I spent a week in New York City, followed by four plane rides in five days, two of which were cross-country flights. Shared air be damned! And I was right –

I was fine. No legitimate scares at all. People told me I was *strong*; that I was a *trooper* and an *inspiration*. I was a fucking idiot.

The thing about wearing a brave face is that your muscles get tired of being on. The physical toll this travel took on my body was crazy, and like clockwork, I would spend the day following travel in bed, barely able to move partially because of fatigue and partially because even the Claritin couldn't help me now.

I was physically and mentally tired to a point that I would sometimes call my mom on my drive to the office in the morning and melt down over the tiniest of details, because when I was alone and in my own head, it was a totally different level of anxiety, exhaustion and doomsday. This was obviously exacerbated by the travel. One morning, I called my mom, progressively breaking into tears because I ran over a lizard. On the highway. In Miami. Ridiculous. Her voice would waver for a minute (I assume she was holding back tears), and then she'd reassure me that I was just tired, and I had the same mini tantrums when I was a kid. "Jess, you just need a nap." (Remember what I said earlier about Forrest Gump? Do it.)

So I'd finish my commute to the office, deal with my morning and then take a 1-hour, lunchtime nap in my car, AC full blast (summers in south Florida are no joke), and then go back inside, eat at my desk and finish the day. Those days usually consisted of comfort food for dinner (read: Farina) and an early bedtime. I'd wake up the following morning to multiple texts and voicemails from my parents checking in on me, worried that I was dead in a gutter. I was fine. I was always fine. And then I was back on a plane.

Thinking back, I can see the details clearly, and because of that, you get this realist's perspective for this chapter of the book; but in that moment, my schedule was exhilarating. It was the most alive I had felt in a long time. Yes, I was tired and weepy and in some physical pain, but what was the alternative? Should I just lay on the couch and watch SportsCenter over and over all day? Would it have been better to succumb to four months of death by boredom and self-pity? I relished in the fact that chemo by way of cancer could kiss my ass. I had not allowed anything or anyone control any aspect of my life since before I moved away to college – and I certainly wasn't going to start at 32. I was living the best life I could, dealing with the consequences and then doing it all over again. I reasoned, "What's the point of fighting so hard to survive if you're not going to live?"

As I mentioned earlier, at first I hadn't set out with any sort of a plan to inspire or be a warrior or change anyone's life. Once I came to terms with *that* term, and changed my attitude, I started to like that people were impressed by the way I was handling everything. That they embraced my Bitmoji and referred to me as Wonder Woman was invigorating. It perpetuated the challenge I bestowed upon myself and fueled my will to win. I was a badass. I was inspiring people by showing them that attitude and fortitude could change the way we deal with difficult situations. Broadway Joe Namath once said, "When you win, nothing hurts." I was winning, but he fibbed.

Too often in life, we require some devastating event to take place before we take a long hard look in the mirror and ask ourselves what is really important, what do we want, what does 'winning' really mean?

Just five years prior, we buried my brother and I had that ah-ha moment: *If not now, when?* New York had given me a new place to live and a new perspective – a fresh perspective – on life. And here I was again... Just like New York, I was having all sorts of new experiences. This time I was travelling to places I had never been, seeing things I had never seen and talking to people I would have otherwise never met. But one toe at a time, I was stepping right back onto that ladder to the top of corporate America. Once again, I became wrapped up in my day-to-day life, going through the motions with my head down, looking at my phone, engaging in the rat race. What took at least a year and a half of being in Manhattan in 2012 took less than 3 months being in Miami in 2017. I was right back in the climb. What the fuck was I doing? All of a sudden, I sure as hell was not winning.

The thing about that spark and ember and flame and blaze I mentioned at the beginning of this chapter is that just like in nature, the fire will ultimately, somehow, someway be extinguished. Maybe you'll die. Maybe you'll be cured.

Either way (or any way in between), the battle concludes, leaving a path of scorched earth in its wake.

Remember what F. Scott Fitzgerald said: "The world only exists in your eyes...you can make it as big or as small as you want." Take your scorched earth and turn it into the foundation upon which you build your new life. And make it as big and as bold and as bad-ass as you want!

CHAPTER
NINETEEN

GOD

God bless the people who deal or come in contact with the people dealing with cancer. Have you noticed it's such a weird and awkward situation. They don't know what to say. They don't know what to do. I'm sure you've gotten or given comments like, "Well, the hardest part is over. Now you heal." Or "God wouldn't give you any challenge you couldn't handle. You'll come through this stronger than ever." I get it, and in some ways, I was (and maybe still am) jealous of their blind faith. It *is* a very difficult, awkward situation; and really, what *are* they supposed to say? I went through cancer and I still don't know what to say to people who are fighting the battle. In all the statements and attempted words of encouragement that I heard, no matter how good the intentions, the religious comments were the ones that really got to me.

I grew up in a fairly strict Catholic household. We went to Church every Sunday, and attended CCD through Confirmation. We 'weren't allowed to date until we were married' and said Grace before dinner. It was the way things were. The way the world worked as far as we knew. And it was fine. Until life started to happen.

I lost my relationship with God when by brother was killed in that motorcycle accident in 2012. I couldn't even go into a church without having flashbacks from the funeral that happened about 65 years too soon, let alone listen to contradictory scripture about "God's plan" and free will. The more I thought about my relationship with God and the Church, the more I started to question and resent the whole institution. Twenty-minute-long homilies about leading a good, honest life and being good and kind to one another then going home to watch football and listen to gossip about everyone we just saw at Mass left me annoyed. Do unto others and all that. Being taught that priests are the conduit to the Almighty and that He speaks through them, but then seeing how they're out there doing all the same things that we're all doing – gossiping, drinking, playing favorites among the congregation; or worse. Not really in His image, is it?

I can honestly say that out of all the Churches I've been to around the world – either as a parishioner or as a visitor – I've personally met and came to know less than a handful of truly holy men. Just a few that I trust enough to believe what they say – that they wouldn't lead me astray, who practice what they preach and seem to believe what they were taught. The others are just really good salesmen.

I say all this looking back, having shed my naivety and taken off those rose-colored glasses. I lost my brother 2 miles from the house, on a day when he wasn't show boating on his motorcycle. He was hit broadside by a 17-year-old girl who may or may not have been texting. Tell me...what part of THE high and mighty plan was this again? Oh, he's in a better place? What's wrong with this place?

But like the proverbial they say, 'time heals all wounds.' And just as things started healing emotionally, spiritually; just as things were going back to this 'new normal' we'd inherited, WHAMMY! Here's your pink ribbon!

Going back to where we started, it was the faith-based comments that irked me. Forgive me in advance for the impending rant.

Really? This was God's plan? What a guy.

Oh yeah? He wouldn't give me anything I couldn't handle? Where the hell is my free will in this situation?

Thanks so much for your prayers. I can feel my incisions healing as you tell me how much you prayed.

You know, the other night I was dead asleep at 6pm and I suddenly woke up feeling amazing. Must have been your prayer.

I know! Those were mean, horrible thoughts that thankfully lived solely in my mind. They were terrible feelings to have when I knew that the person saying them really meant well; that they simply didn't know what to say and were just trying to make me feel better… but still, they were there (cue *Phantom of the Opera* soundtrack). So on top of feeling like shit physically, I started to feel like an asshole. Wonderful. Please tell me you're empathizing at least a little bit here…

Some people have a theory that you put your faith in God because when you know he has your back, you're never going through anything alone. That sounds nice. That sounds like a fairy tale. I mean, who wouldn't want to believe that, if for no other reason than to fill some void or fear of going through life alone?

But let's play this out, shall we? I have free will. YES. My decisions are mine. YES. All the time. ALL THE TIME. Read the Good book. Go to church. Live a sin-free, meaningful life. YOU GOT IT. So…If I choose correctly, it was God's plan? YES. But, if I choose (via my free will) or do or say something wrong…that's also God's plan? YES. So I have free will, but it actually doesn't mean anything because no matter what I choose, it was already part of His plan? PRETTY MUCH. ONE TIIIIINY THING THOUGH…

IF YOU CHOOSE WRONG – OR IF YOU DON'T CONFESS FOR THAT WRONG THING – THAT 'SIN,' YOU'RE GOING TO HELL. Oh.

So, rules and fear of punishment. Why am I here again? Oh, right – so I'm not alone. But what if I'm kind of okay being alone? Welcome to Catholicism! Here's your free will; enjoy! #DamnedIfYouDo #DamnedIfYouDont

But you know what, none of that even matters. Because I was bought in. From birth, really. Maybe that's what made it worse when I got my diagnosis. I went to church on more than just Christmas and Easter. I was the good kid and prayed. I obeyed my parents: no underage drinking; no drugs; no smoking. I played by the rules for the most part, and when I didn't, I went to Confession. I did as they said, not as they did. I was a good person, lived by the golden rule...everything. So where did cancer come from? Not my genes. Not bad habits. No explanation! What part of the plan was this?

I slowly began to eliminate dogmatic parts of Catholicism from my life. I no longer went to Church on Sundays. I no longer crossed myself before Grace, or even said Grace before meals. I didn't say anything like "So sorry for your loss. Thoughts and prayers are with you and your family." It simply became 'thoughts.' People would say they prayed for me and that they asked God for blessings in my favor; and I'd smile politely and thank them, but honestly, it meant nothing.

It was such a hard time. Really seeing no value in these principles and beliefs I had been raised on, like 30 years of teachings were for nothing... It's not that I didn't believe in God. That was never a question – the universe is too expansive; and science is too perfect for there not to be a higher power; but I was mad. And sad. And maybe a bit petulant. But I got over that part. You want to know why? Because this was *my* battle. And *my* body. And I was allowed to feel however the fuck *I* wanted to feel. It was no one's place to tell me how I *should* feel or how I *should* deal with this situation or to turn to God for answers and guidance. For me, God had done enough already.

Whether you have been diagnosed, or are supporting someone who has, remember that. You get to feel how you want and do whatever it takes to survive – mentally, physically and spiritually – and if that means you do it with or without your God, or some mix in between, it's your prerogative. And supporters, since your patient likely won't say anything to you directly (they have enough going on), I'll say it for them: There is no time for lectures or opinions, and they probably don't want to hear it anyway. Take your soapbox elsewhere or save it for the pulpit. If and/or when they want your guidance on this matter, trust me – they'll ask for it.

CHAPTER
TWENTY

BE KIND

Going through cancer taught me so much. In some cases, it taught me life lessons that I'll forever cherish. In other cases, it taught me about Biology, Physiology and all the other '-ology's. Sometimes, it even taught me about perspective – both mine and that of other people. Probably the most profound though, was what it taught me about myself and self-awareness.

For a long time, there was meme circulating that spoke to our inability to know what other people are going through at any given moment. It seems to pop up again every time there's a new label for or case of bullying, or a terrible event that takes place that rocks society. The message was to be kind, no matter what, as you never know what someone else is dealing with. I liked it. It seemed logical so at some point I'm sure I pinned and shared it for all the world to see.

Before cancer, I equated the sentiment with pertaining to mental health issues, or someone having just been fired or laid off from their job; maybe a bad breakup or domestic abuse. As a result of seeing it through that lens, I associated it with the general concept of not being a jerk to strangers. A very deliberate decision to or not to say something ignorant, mean, sarcastic or insensitive.

It was not until I went through this journey and experienced certain situations for myself that I really understood it on a deeper level. Sure, words, phrases, general sentiments are important; and we should always be cognizant of the way we present ourselves to those who don't know our cultural colloquialisms or personal quirks; but it goes so far beyond speech and syntax:

Body language, facial ticks and twinges.

Staring, or purposely not staring.

Whispers and hushed tones (they are never as hushed as you think they are)

The word cancer itself.

Snide comments and opinions.

General topics of conversation.

Our society in America, which is chock-full of loud opinions and unsolicited advice, can be a pretty rough place – especially if you don't look like everyone else. At one point after my third chemo treatment, once I had lost all my luscious locks and was rocking the cue ball style, which is usually socially reserved for middle-aged men, I was walking through the mall in Miami. This mall was buzzing with people of all sorts of backgrounds – some white, some Latino, some black, some brown…a good mixture. I was doing my thing, not thinking about much of anything aside from the (probably) sweatpants I needed to buy, when I tuned in to the passing strollers and toddlers holding their mothers' hands. The children would look at me curiously. *How strange*, I could read on their faces, *that person looks like a woman (my mommy carries a purse) and has makeup on… but she has no hair… like daddy.* They'd fixate for a moment, seemingly trying to figure it out, come to some sort of terms with what they were seeing, comprehend to whatever degree and then move on, learning and experiencing the next frame of life to cross their paths.

Children are so innocent, so pure and so unabashedly curious, yet understanding. Their parents were different. I could feel the glance from 50 feet away. I could read their faces: *Oh shit, she looks weird. Must be really sick. Quick, look away! Don't make eye contact, you don't want to seem like you're staring. C'mere honey, stay far away from the obviously contagious woman, who has something wrong with her.* It thickens your skin. It also makes you want to punch them in the throat.

I had purchased a wig, had it fitted and trimmed to my liking, and it looked fine. However, during my chemo sessions, I was living in Miami. It was summer; it was around 90 degrees outside, and it was quite a process to put this wig on and keep looking good all day. Maybe I could have avoided situations like this, but why should I have to?

We all have a look. You know the look I'm referring to. It's the one where your face contorts unintentionally and without your consent when you see something you disapprove of. An all-too-trendy teenager, a mismatched suit and tie combo, over the top makeup…You know the look (you probably just inadvertently made that look) and I'm here to bestow some of my newfound self-awareness on you: that look does more harm than you probably realize. Do me, yourself and everyone you know a favor: sit in front of a mirror and think of cringe-worthy phrases and outfits or actions that bother you. Watch your automatic reactions and work on keeping a poker face. Do this exercise again and again until your face doesn't give away your oh-so-private internal monologue.

* * *

One afternoon pre-cancer, I was with some friends when a surprisingly civil, albeit thorough conversation about women breastfeeding babies in public broke out. Tangentially, we spoke about whether we would breastfeed our own children should the need for such a decision ever present itself, the alternative being formula bottle feeding. We shared our opinions, thoughts and feelings over what was most likely a boozy brunch. Some were very set in one camp or another, but we all respected each other's views and had a nice conversation. I'm lucky and proud to have very intelligent, opinionated and reasonable friends, but it's not lost on me how sideways a conversation like this could have gone.

Since that point in time, my perspective has changed...Imagine if my friends and I had been walking through a park and saw a woman bottle-feeding her young child. *How unnatural*, some of us might think. What if this were you? Would you turn to your friend and begin to have a conversation similar to the one my friends and I had over brunch, paying no mind to your proximity to this woman and her child. Would you talk about how *your* babies were breastfed and how that's the way it's supposed to be done? *After all, God wouldn't have given us the ability to sustain our offspring if we were meant to bottle feed.* How Christian of you.

What you don't know is that that woman used the last two of her frozen eggs to barely get pregnant at the age of 37. She froze them when she was 32, right before undergoing Chemotherapy after a double mastectomy. She and her husband had planned to travel for a while and enjoy each other's company before taking the plunge into parenthood – and once they finally reached the point where they started exploring the possibility of children, she was hit with a pink wall of reality. She actually no longer has the physical ability to breastfeed her child – something she had looked forward to since she got married ten years ago. She's lucky she was even able to get pregnant at all, after Chemo wiped out her natural ability to do so. Now she's four years behind on her plan, she's barely maintaining her composure thanks to her new normal and she has a newborn…while getting hot flashes because menopause set in 15 years earlier than expected. What if, on top of all that, she was doing the whole thing on her own, without a significant other? Good thing you shared your opinion, huh?

I found myself all of a sudden remarkably more aware of situations like this, because aside from never having really analyzed my own views on certain circumstances (breastfeeding being one of them), I may very well have been the one obnoxiously sharing my opinion, not even thinking about the reasons behind that woman's decision (not that she needs a reason, for the record). Is this a true story? Does it matter? You get my point. These days, I constantly remind myself, "Don't be a jerk – self-righteous isn't cute on anyone."

* * *

In my corporate roles, I've come across a term used for a person or group within a team or company who do more harm than good. They have bad attitudes, low tolerance and are constant complainers. They're usually not very good at their jobs either. We refer to them as a *cancer*. We talk about them as if they are a festering collection of bad ideas, bad energy and bad blood, put wherever they are just to make us miserable – to make our jobs harder. And cancers don't just exist in the workplace. Maybe you have a cancer in your life – a mooching family member, or a friend that never quite grew up like the rest of you. What if you are the cancer in your group?

Be honest – how many times did you wince, reading that paragraph? I've certainly used this phrasing before, and now it hurts my fingers to type. In all fairness, though, the descriptor is right on – it is literally the perfect term for what it's intending to describe. That's not to say it's not incredibly insensitive to anyone who has been diagnosed or who is very close to someone who has. What if you're using that word in that context in a conversation with someone who has recently been diagnosed, but hasn't yet told anyone? How would you feel if you were in his or her situation? What is the implied context to this group of people you're referring to as a cancer? Did they cost you in excess of one hundred thousand dollars? Did they cost you months, maybe years of your life? Did they cost you your mind, body, maybe your soul? Did they change your life, your perspective forever? Did they cost you the life of a loved one?

And what do we do about those cancers anyway? It would make sense that rather than bitching and moaning about said cancer, management would simply manage the person or group out, or better yet just let them go – a management mastectomy...but that never happens, does it? How do you address the cancers in your life? You certainly don't call them a cancer…or do you? Maybe you do…How does that go over?

I'm not saying that any word which carries multiple meanings should never be used in the other context, or that you should walk on eggshells; but if you're not going to do anything about the situation, what's the point of highlighting it using such a stinging term?

* * *

Post-cancer, my self-awareness is on high alert. I imagine you'll relate to some of these thoughts moving forward, but if not, that's cool too. Just like my learning that you know your body better than anyone else, you also are the master of your domain. You can think what you want, say what you want and phrase your words however you want, but my role in all of this is to share my experiences and learnings. So here you go: Outside of specific conversations with social acceptances among the group, no one cares about your opinion on breastfeeding versus bottle feeding. Everything that is bad is not automatically a cancer. Until you have had cancer, please don't equate a bad attitude or sub-par professional performance to the thing that has rocked so many people's worlds. Nobody wants to know if you think my tits are real or fake – and it is none of your God-damned business. Your opinion on my bald head, my sunken eyes, my scars can go jump in a lake. It's not fun for you to play with my breasts during foreplay because I have no reaction? That's because I can't actually feel anything you're doing. Where are my nipples? In a bio-waste dump somewhere, probably. Oh, this is awkward? Welcome to my world.

All that said, you don't have to be a stick in the mud as you go through treatments. Like I said before, find the opportunities to laugh, because there's no doubt there will be a lot of reasons to cry! We had gone to visit my grandparents and some of my mom's side of the family in Sebastian, Florida for Easter of 2017. This #SeasonalSelfie was one of my favorites, as me, my dad and my brother-in-law were all bald at the time (they still are). To celebrate, the three of us painted Easter eggs on our heads, and my mom and sister were Easter bunnies. It was so much fun and provided such a reprieve from thinking about cancer! We didn't have a chance to wash off the paint before some of the other guests arrived for dinner, and as I said hello and hugged my cousin, Michael[10], he jumped back, and ever so eloquently yelled, "Ugh! You're sweaty and you're bald!" The room screeched to a halt. Everyone clenched their teeth, biting their top and bottom lips at the same time, waiting for my reaction before sharing theirs. I had not belly laughed so hard in such a long time…They joined in and it's a now a running joke with the family.

Regardless of your thoughts on any or all of those topics, I don't think there are too many people in this world that would fight me on the thought that we need to get to a place where we are kinder to one another. There's a

[10] Michael has Downs Syndrome, is extremely animated and has zero filter.

saying in business: Two ears, one mouth. Normally in business, people say this when speaking to or about salespeople. Listen more, talk less. In the context of cancer and, more generally, being a good person, compassion, empathy, kindness, understanding, giving, caring…Those are our ears. Our mouths are our actions and our words. If we listen and observe more and shoot our mouths off less, the world would be a much better place for everyone. Do your part and inspire others to do theirs.

CHAPTER
TWENTY-ONE

GRIEF

As you go through your journey, there will likely be people along the way who ask you how you're handling the situation, and once you move through the very obvious physical part, will start to use the word, 'grief.' When I first hit this recovery milestone, the one where people – no matter their emotional closeness to you – start to ask questions that are maybe just a little too personal, I didn't really know how to answer them. As far as I was concerned, I didn't need to grieve. Looking back, I equate this to the sentiment regarding self-breast exams. Humor me for a moment... Do you remember how your doctors or Sex Ed teachers would tell you to make sure you're checking your breasts in the shower, or wherever? I remember thinking, *What is a lump even going to feel like? How would I know if it's cancer or not? This is stupid.* But then, years later when I felt *my* lump, I knew exactly what they were talking about. When you know, you know, right? Well, I came to realize that the reason I couldn't answer the questions about grief was because I hadn't grieved yet.

Though totally normal, and what I've come to realize is a really important step in the journey, grief can sneak up on you. I doubt anyone sets out specifically to grieve. I know I didn't just sit down on the couch one day and tell myself, "Ok, today I'll grieve." But all of a sudden, out of nowhere and usually at the most inopportune time, grief hits you like a truck.

One commonly accepted grief process is the Klüber-Ross Cycle, which includes five steps: Denial, Anger, Depression, Bargaining and Acceptance. It's widely accepted as well that these steps are neither equally distributed, nor carry the same duration; and sometimes, not everyone experiences all five of these steps in the cycle. In short, everyone grieves differently.

In my case, this happened right after my final chemo session.

When they pulled the needle from my port and bandaged me up, I instantly felt lighter. I felt strong and weak in the same moment. It was over and for the first time in five months, I truly exhaled. There were no decisions to be made, no next steps to re-arrange my schedule for…just a moment to breathe.

I didn't have to put on a brave face anymore. I didn't have to be positive and will my way through the process. I could just be. And cry. And rest. I grabbed my balloons and all my chemo supplies, most of which hadn't been used, bid adieu to the nurses and doctors and walked out of the building with my parents in tow. I couldn't get out of there fast enough, but it was also surprisingly hard to leave. On one hand, this was a *wait, that's it?* moment; but on the other hand, I never wanted to see any of these people ever again…

Once outside, I took the obligatory selfie and suddenly I saw myself the way others saw me. For the first time in five months, I raised the veil of control and saw my sunken, dark eyes, my obviously-penciled-on eyebrows, my gray skin. I noticed that my eyes had changed color a bit – they were darker – and my fingernails were grossly thin and flaky. I had gained a ton of weight and my hands and feet tingled from neuropathy. I had bags under my eyes, I was pale and the little bit of my hair that was trying to come back was feathery and sparse – like an old man who wasn't ready to come to terms with his impending baldness. I *looked* sick.

Had I been in denial this whole time? Had I convinced myself that every day since February was just another day in paradise? Was this a coping mechanism or the first step of grief rearing its ugly head? As I sit and reflect now, I don't think it was any of those things. In my never-have-I-ever-gone-to-medical-school opinion, this was simply a lack of time and emotional capacity to see things the way they truly were... Part of the compartmentalization we talked about earlier. Maybe it was self-preservation. Maybe I didn't have time to care about something so trivial as my appearance as I was fighting for my life. Maybe I didn't want to see it. No matter how you look at it (see what I did there?) choosing to see myself without the veil would not have done anyone any good through the process. Besides, denial set in later.

Not all of these stages of grief will be dramatic or clear. For me, most of them came pretty quickly. They seem to have been bottled up inside for five months, and as I did my "Last Chemo" live stream, they all came pouring out of my mouth like verbal diarrhea.

I couldn't believe that it was over – or that it had even begun, and because the entire experience had been such a rapid fire of events, decisions and appointments, I had never taken the time to even think about the whole ordeal, let alone deal with it on an emotional level. I cried, but I kept rolling.

I was mad that I had to deal with the entire situation at all. Angry that I had done everything right and yet, here I was. I was pissed off that I had to have implants, and that I had to go through menopause. I was livid that everything from here on out was going to be more difficult. I still had another surgery ahead of me, which meant more time off work, more medication, more money, more healing, more drains, fucking drains. I didn't like that people knew about my cancer and that my identity would ultimately revolve around the worst seven months of my life. How unfair it was that I might not be able to have kids, and worse that these scars would forever haunt my self-image. I was angry with my body; I was mad at God; and I was livid with the decisions I had made in the past.

When people talk about grief and the stages in the grief cycle, it's easy to discount the concept if you haven't experienced it for yourself. It's very easy to scoff at the process and be skeptical that there's even a need to codify the whole ordeal. I was one of those people. I didn't see grief as a weakness per se, but I always thought it was a little bit dramatic. *Just deal with your shit and let me know when you're good to get back to normal. Cool?* Of course, I never said this out loud, but if I'm being truly honest with myself, it was in my head. For what it's worth, I did this to myself as well. The thing is, you don't recognize grief as it's happening, but rather it comes to light in retrospect as you think to yourself, "What the fuck was that?!"

Anger devolved into depression, and I found myself overthinking all the things I was mad at and about. If only I hadn't waited to report the lump – maybe this would have only been a small surgery. (Nope.) What if I hadn't focused so much on my career, then maybe I would already be married and had a kid; and I wouldn't have to worry about [insert laundry list here]. (Also, nope.) If…. If… If… It's a vicious cycle and one that spirals lower and lower the longer you're in it, and sometimes it takes a little bit of tough love to get out. Maybe that tough love comes from a friend or a parent; maybe it comes from a therapist; maybe it comes from within. The important part to remember is that it's normal; it's okay not to be okay; and this too shall pass.

I don't remember a specific phase of bargaining, but there were definitely times that I thought to myself, "Once this is over, I'm going to be more active, go out and meet new people, or spend more time with my loved ones." "As soon as I get my new boobs, and this is 100% behind me, that's it – a new leaf!"

This didn't last too long before I slapped some sense into myself and decided to accept things for what they were. I was faced with adversity, I took care of business, and I lived to tell the tale. *Suck it up, Buttercup (that's me). It's over, let's move on.*

I've come to believe that acceptance truly is as simple as making the decision to accept the situation, but it's also undoubtedly the most difficult step. The way I see it, your entire life is really just a series of decisions: Am I going to have a good day or a bad day? Chicken or Steak? Coke or water? Be nasty or nice? Sarcastic or helpful? Share this post or realize not everyone needs to be exposed to my unfiltered, inner monologue? Are we happy or sad today? When something bad happens…will I own it or let it own me?

The absolute toughest question I had to answer for myself during the grieving process was *Am I going to let cancer define me?* Initially, the answer was a hard no. And I fought it. God, I fought it so hard. I tried to act as though none of this had ever happened; that those three years of my life were something out of a telenovela and I was the one with amnesia. I was determined to pick up where I left off prior to the diagnosis and charge on like it never happened. Like I hadn't had two massive surgeries and been through chemotherapy and everything that came with that. Like I hadn't dreaded the time in between my six-month check-ins with the doctors because *what if it's back?* Like I hadn't been fundamentally changed forever after being forced to consider the alternative to surviving. Cancer was not going to define me. Cancer would not be the thing people thought of first when hearing my name or meeting me. I was not a victim of cancer and as far as cancer and I were concerned, we were done, over, kaput.

But people knew about my cancer, and they were interested in hearing about the story. They wanted to share it with other people in their respective networks that they thought would benefit. I couldn't escape this time in my life, no matter how hard I tried. Even when I joined Toastmasters, despite promising myself I wouldn't cite this period of my life, I found myself drawing on my experiences with cancer to give merit to my thoughts and declarations; and even at work, I went back to 2017 in my mind to help keep my emotions and points of view in check when dealing with the human side of business. The fight against cancer changed my perspective and made me more aware of what's really important, how certain circumstances and instances weigh against one another in the grand scheme of life and gave context to not sweating the small stuff. ("Small" is relative, by the way.)

Hard as I tried, and as often as I told myself I was, the truth is that I wasn't content or settled on this new, *Cancer-won't-define-me* mindset. Something was missing from my logic – it wasn't working. Before long, I retreated a bit and forced myself to consider what 'being defined by cancer' really meant. If I could help others with my story, or use this less-than-favorable predicament to my benefit, why not? Historically, I had used all my other life experiences as needed, without thinking twice. Why should this be any different? From that day, I made a conscious effort to embrace my cancer journey and take control of the story. Rather than leaving it up to others to spring on me, I could take it upon myself to own it and use it and thrive even more because of it. This plan started to work. I was getting more comfortable talking about it, more confident in using it for good and my life was seeming to settle.

The day I was officially *CURED*, I decided to finally and truly **accept** cancer for the role it would play in my day-to-day life moving forward. My mind was suddenly more at peace than it had been in three years. I stopped fighting against the ghost that was cancer and was able to channel my energy and anxiety into more productive feats.

Your mind is a powerful thing, but there will be times during this journey that it will play tricks on you. It will forget things and it will make you feel somewhat illiterate and it will give you strength you didn't know you had. It will make you feel 100% exposed one minute and invincible the next. It will numb you to things you've feared for your entire life, empower you to see things clearer than ever before and make you raise your bar on so many levels. The mind is so impressive. Let it do its thing but keep it in check and don't let it overwhelm you.

CHAPTER
TWENTY-TWO

PERSPECTIVE

I've talked a lot about attitude and grief and acceptance, and throughout those discussions, perspective has been a common thread. According to Webster, perspective is a noun that means "a particular way of viewing something; a point of view." According to yours truly, it is the quintessential combination of what some people refer to as being both a blessing and a curse...and also what Webster said. Perspective is a culmination of our opinions about our experiences in life and a hodge-podge of lessons learned – for better or worse.

Similar to the point when you decide you're ready to ride without training wheels, have your first kiss or talk openly with your parents about how much you drank in college, there's a tipping point in perspective: the point where you decide that your perspective is solid enough to verbalize it. You've seen, heard and done enough to be confident in the point of view you're about to express, you're well equipped enough to defend any feedback, and you're enlightened enough to adapt should your perspective be met with one you agree with more than your own.

I've found perspective to be a double-edged sword. In some ways, it is a blessing that guides us through life, dynamically pivoting and adjusting by taking into account the layers of experience as we add to our lens along the way. It incites empathy, gives clarity to otherwise muddy waters and allows us to keep a running scale of *it could be worse*. On the flip side, perspective can cloud our judgment and not let us see the beauty in the simplicity of life. Having been through *too much*, we may find it difficult to bask in the moment, no matter how small or seemingly insignificant.

That second side of perspective can be a dark one – one that I've come to realize is very difficult to overcome. After losing my brother and subsequently getting diagnosed with cancer, going through treatments and managing the waiting game, I sometimes find myself numb to the emotions and feelings of other people. As I fought and fought to maintain my attitude-as-an-asset, I occasionally retreated into a place where it was difficult for me to empathize with people who freaked out over menial (to me) daily occurrences or who had a hard time making seemingly unimportant (to me) decisions, or who couldn't cope with the loss of a irrelevant (to me) popstar. After all, if you haven't lost a brother or dealt with cancer, or lost your grandpa a month before your final chemo session, have you even a right to be sad? I mean, in the grand scheme of things, what they were going through wasn't really that bad, was it? *Holy shit, Jessica! When did you become such an asshole?*

I found myself saying that often: *in the grand scheme...* But whose grand scheme were we even talking about? And where did I get off having these opinions, let alone vocalizing them to anyone? I knew this was not the right sentiment, and that opinions like those were unnecessary and did more harm than good.

To this day though, I find myself overly sensitive and having next to zero patience for people who, in my opinion, take certain things (like family relationships, illness, etc.) for granted, or who are completely unreasonable in their perspectives. When thoughts like these enter my head, I usually try to keep them to myself; however, I'm still working on *that look* we talked about earlier, and it's not quite yet perfected. When my expressions get away from me, and someone notices and asks about it, I'm happy to oblige them with my thoughts (since they asked), but these days, I'm more equipped to use some tact, present these thoughts in an ironclad way on the fly and make my point succinctly.

I have a confession: I lied. Perspective way worse than the double-edged sword I called it earlier. It's actually more of a multi-dimensional worm hole with lots of different angles, clarity points, sharp edges and blunt-force trauma. In early summer 2017, I was having a normal, daily conversation with a colleague (turned friend) at the office. In typical cadence, we asked each other how we were doing. He was obviously under the weather, and I told him that he should have stayed home. He said, "How can I justify staying home because of a cold when you haven't taken one day off during chemo?"

What a horrible feeling, his perspective of my perspective. Here I was, coming to work for the sole purpose of staying sane and staying distracted from my reality, and he saw it as some sort of challenge, a bar set to the highest level. It made me realize that perspective is a living, breathing, changing, adapting organism – a constant pivot point. I thought about what he said for a moment and responded, "My being here the day after chemo in no way diminishes you not feeling well. It's all relative. I'm sicker than you are, so you're not sick enough for it to matter? Maybe we should both go home!" We chuckled, uncomfortably, and went on with our days.

I originally started this book right after my reconstruction in 2017 (approximately seven and a half months after diagnosis) and it sat at about 1500 words in my OneDrive for two years before I was able to finish. I hesitated for a while because I hadn't yet dealt with that curse of perspective. Here I am now, 3 ½ years outside of diagnosis, wiser and more eloquent than ever, and I can finally put into words what I couldn't back then, when my co-worker enlightened me.

Do not compare yourself to others.

Your situation in life – no matter how seemingly insignificant – is important, valid and worthy all on its own.

There is no scorecard, but if you do it right, everybody wins.

One of my favorite movies is *Little Giants*, a youth football-centric underdog story, starring Rick Moranis and Ed O'Neil, that showcases the fallout of sibling rivalry, the power of believing in yourself and the brilliant strategy of the *Annexation of Puerto Rico*.

In the case of the two adult brothers in this movie, it's important to note that the older brother (O'Neil's character) is a retired NFL player who had been extremely 'successful' in the league and now runs the small Ohio town's largest auto dealership. He has a huge house, seems to want for nothing and has three doting females in his life (a wife and two daughters). The younger brother, played by Moranis, owns and operates the local gas station/body shop. He is a single dad (wife passed away) who is raising a tom-boy-ish daughter all on his own. They have a modest life and in contrast to his brother, is what you might call frumpy.

There's a scene in the movie where Ed O'Neil's character drives up next to his (walking) brother (Rick Moranis) in a sick convertible and starts a one-sided conversation. At the end of the conversation, before Moranis can respond, O'Neil says, "I knew you'd see it my way." He speeds off, leaving Moranis befuddled, but not shocked by the interaction. Status quo, so it seems.

I'll save you the spoiler, but later on in the plot, at a very strategic point, where the score crescendos, Ed repeats this line to his brother; and for seemingly the first time in his life, Rick Moranis grows a pair and replies, "You know what? I don't see it your way. In fact, I've never seen it your way!" He completes his thought and the story continues to its all-too-foreseeable conclusion, but we're left with the feeling of victory. In that moment, Moranis' character expressed his perspective and he (and those around him) were better off for it.

The different experiences of the underdog team (personified for simplicity in Moranis' character) didn't mean that they were less important than the favorites. Their smaller-than-the-opponent stature didn't automatically seal their fate as being losers. The older, stronger, wiser voice's decision to offer their perspective doesn't automatically mean you have to accept it as-is. The Giants had every right to share the field with the Cowboys and use their collective experiences – their perspective – to play the game. Watch the movie. You won't be disappointed.

You need to feel your feelings, and to express them. To have your perspective influence and impact the way you experience events, conversations and interactions in life is what makes us human and productive members of society. What you do or say, or how you act in the context of your perspective is how we all learn from one another and grow together.

Let me ask you a question… Do you know anyone who has had the exact same life experiences that you have? Like, exact? Your perspective – be it as a warrior, as a survivor or as a supporter – is forever changed. There is no going back to Before Cancer. It doesn't exist anymore. As Taylor Swift said, "I'm sorry, the old Taylor can't come to the phone right now. Why? Oh, 'cause she's dead." Before Cancer YOU is dead.

Take all the experiences you had pre-cancer and archive them somewhere in an easily accessible part of your chemo brain. From now on, you'll see things through the lens of After Cancer. The world is brand new to your new perspective – one that has received (likely) the worst news of your life and lived to tell about it. One that has been poked and prodded and cut open and sewn back up. One that decided to fight. One that decided keep fighting. One that wasn't ashamed to ask for help. One that looked mortality in the face and told it to fuck off. One that found the strength to continue on.

CHAPTER
TWENTY-THREE

STRENGTH

In this world on its own, let alone when you deal with something like cancer, it's sometimes hard to realize – and subsequently remember – just how strong you are. Hopefully this will remind you.

My friend, you are and will forever be better equipped than you think you are. You have a mind and a heart all your own. You take no shit from anyone and you forge your own path. You wake up each morning and you live your life – your best life. Every day is different – you're adaptable. You expect the unexpected, dream the unimaginable and ride waves others wouldn't even attempt.

You are strong.

You think about things before anyone else thinks about them. You lift others up and applaud greatness. You embody powerful, incite excellence and emanate grace. You're smart, concerted and excitable. You find hope when there is none, you exude confidence when you're unsure and you breathe life into otherwise expired situations.

You are powerful.

You're creative and cunning. Sharp as a tack and smart as a whip. You're nimble and quick and you manage the impossible. You're lighthearted and funny, but serious and steadfast. You laugh at yourself and respect others. You strive to be the best version of yourself and you are succeeding.

You are a force to be reckoned with.

You are territorial and protective with the best of intentions. You know your mind, body and soul and you're not afraid to share yourself – your whole self – with the world. Because what a disgrace it would be for you to hide. You bring tremendous value. You can do anything you put your mind to and there is nothing that could ever, would ever or should ever get in your way.

You are a strong, powerful force to be reckoned with.

You, my dear, are a WARRIOR.

Here's to strong women.

May we know them. May we be them.
May we raise them.

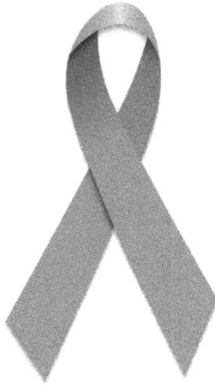

#CancerSucks

ACKNOWLEDGEMENTS

It goes without saying that my parents are number one on the list of people that I owe the success of this book to. Without them, their support and their willingness to be present during my journey, I'm not sure I would have made it through at all, let alone in such good spirits. Aside from the support they gave me during the worst seven months of my life, they raised me to be a strong, independent woman. They told me I could do anything, be anything and conquer anything I put my mind to. I'm so lucky to have had their love and guidance, and even more so to have inherited the perfect balance of their wit, wherewithal and moxie.

To the friends and family who were along for the ride from a distance through Jess's Cancer Fighting Squad, your support and encouragement was something that I didn't realize I would need as much as I did. Between the kind words, constant reassurance and funny and heartfelt memes and texts you sent or posted, I can't tell you how much love I felt, and in turn was able to use to push through the tough days. Even by just tuning into my live videos, or watching them later, I never felt alone and was constantly reminded about what I was fighting for.

To the doctors, staff and administrators that were involved in my journey, thank you for making it so bearable and for bringing the bits of levity when needed. Oh yeah, and for getting this cancer out of me.

I couldn't have gotten through cancer, let alone written this book if I didn't have a Rockstar group of very close friends to keep me sane, grounded and pushing through. When I needed to curse and vent and lose my mind, you were there to listen. When I needed you to kick me in the ass a bit, you were there with a loving touch. When I was being a bit ridiculous, you kept me in check. I look forward to growing old with you!

For almost two years, my grandma was the only one who saw any portion of the manuscript for WARRIOR, and her encouragement and desire to keep reading helped push me over the finish line. Thank you for your faith in me, your discretion and for your support through the (extremely long and drawn out) writing process. So you know, I brought the *f*ck* count from 29 to 23 (that one doesn't count).

To all of you who got this far, thank you for reading about my journey and I hope to God you just wanted to read something different. If you do happen to be fighting cancer, I hope this helped you and your supporters! You have my thoughts, (more recently) prayers and support, 110%. You can and will beat this!

RESOURCES

For resources, videos and more, visit:

FACEBOOK.COM/WARRIORGUIDEBOOK

AND

WWW.WARRIORGUIDEBOOK.COM

www.ingramcontent.com/pod-product-compliance
Lightning Source LLC
Chambersburg PA
CBHW071422270326
41914CB00042BB/2056/J